The Joint Health
PRESCRIPTION

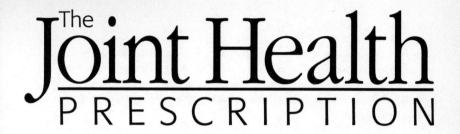

The Joint Health PRESCRIPTION

8 Weeks to Stronger, Healthier, Younger Joints

James M. Rippe, M.D.

with Sean McCarthy, M.S., and Mary Abbott Waite, Ph.D.

BALLANTINE BOOKS • NEW YORK

Internet addresses and telephone numbers given in this book were accurate
at the time the book went to press.

The research study upon which this book is based was funded in part by a grant
from Nabisco, Inc.

A Ballantine Book
Published by The Ballantine Publishing Group
Copyright © 2001 by James M. Rippe

www.ballantinebooks.com

Library of Congress Control Number: 2002113793

ISBN 0-345-45117-1

This edition published by arrangement with Rodale Inc.

Cover design by Mike Stromberg
Cover photo © Bob Kraemer/Index Stock Imagery

Manufactured in the United States of America

First Ballantine Books Edition: December 2002

1 3 5 7 9 10 8 6 4 2

To Stephanie, Hart, Jaelin, and Devon
The fire and the rose are one . . .

CONTENTS

Part III: The Joint Owner's Maintenance Manual

Resources

ACKNOWLEDGMENTS

Both research and book writing are collaborative efforts. It is not possible to cite all of the individuals who have contributed to the research project and to this book. However, I would like to single out some individuals for their special contributions.

First, my main collaborator, Mary Abbott Waite, Ph.D. Mary Abbott is a fantastic writing partner. She took a scientific manuscript and shaped it into the coherent, motivational book that you will have the pleasure of reading. Mary Abbott and I have worked together on numerous books. She is simply the best! Not only is she a wonderful writer, she also contributes numerous important insights and makes a major contribution to the scientific underpinnings of these projects.

Sean McCarthy, M.S., has been a hard-working and highly valued exercise physiologist in my laboratory in Shrewsbury, Massachusetts, the Rippe Lifestyle Institute (RLI). Sean not only led our study on joint health on a day-to-day basis but also contributed in very meaningful ways to the final shape and content of this manuscript, particularly in coordinating development of the self-tests and exercise programs for the 8-Week Joint Health Program.

My editorial director and good friend Beth Porcaro guided the entire project with her usual blend of good humor and superb organizational skills.

Many scientists at RLI contributed to the study. This scientific team is led by my friend and colleague Kyle McInnis, Sc.D., who provides not only superb scientific insight and direction to all of our endeavors but also collaborates on every scientific project that emanates from our laboratory. For this project, he shared his expertise in clinical exercise physiology to assist in the creation of the strength-training program. Michael Carpenter, M.S., a staff exercise physiologist, worked extensively on the study. He also provided excellent insight into the exercise programs used in this book. Our rheumatology consultant, Eric Jacobson, M.D., guided the development of the book's medical assessment chapter. Maren Fragala, B.S, a summer intern for RLI, spent many hours in the library obtaining copies of the original research used to develop this book. Our former director of marketing and communication, Amy Myrdal, M.S., R.D., lent her extensive expertise to developing the nutrition and supplement chapters. Senior scientist Kathleen Melanson, R.D., Ph.D.; staff exercise physiologists Jason Gootman, M.S., C.S.C.S., and Will Kirousis, B.S., C.S.C.S.; dietitians Dina Berlin, R.D., M.S., and Jessica Dell'Olio, R.D., M.S.; staff nurse Sandi Knipe, R.N., B.S.N.; and athletic trainer Jennifer Barry, B.S., A.T.C., were great assets in answering questions or critiquing when necessary.

Special praise is due to the more than 200 men and women who participated in the study, who showed tremendous dedication and enthusiasm for the project. Participation was very time-consuming and arduous. Each subject had to report to our laboratory a minimum of 18 times over a 14-week period. Without the participants' enthusiasm and hard work, the study could never have been done.

Help in shaping the initial concept for this book came from my friend and literary agent, Reid Boates, along with Tami Booth, executive editor of Women's Health Books at Rodale. Both Tami and Reid have collaborated with me on a number of other books. Their expertise, friendship, and enthusiasm are highly valued. I would also like to acknowledge the valuable contribution of Nabisco, Inc., and the Knox Company, which supported the research behind this book.

Many of the clinical insights in this book are employed on a daily basis at my clinical facility. My wonderful staff at Rippe Health Assessment (RHA) at Celebration Health in Celebration, Florida—including Chris Young, R.N., clinic manager; Rick Wassel, director of sales and marketing; Sara McCoy, my executive assistant at RHA; Page Sturgill, manager of client services; Joan Clarke, R.N.; Holly Bell; and Tara Geise, R.D., M.S.—have all provided important insights and ongoing clinical validation of many of the concepts discussed in this book.

My complex life, including responsibilities and commitments as a cardiologist, researcher, writer, consultant, and teacher, sometimes seems to require a magician to make all these activities mesh into one schedule. My executive assistant at RLI, Carol Moreau, does a phenomenal job of keeping these strands of my life intertwined and the entire endeavor moving forward. I am indebted to her for her competence, good humor, and caring.

Last, but certainly not least, my darling wife and lifelong partner,

Stephanie Hart Rippe, provides me with love, support, and security, without which none of this would be possible or worthwhile. She supports my intense work schedule and inspires me daily with her love, courage, competence, beauty, and intelligence. In addition, she has given me three beautiful daughters, Hart Elizabeth Rippe, Jaelin Davis Rippe, and Devon Marshall Rippe. These are the four beautiful "Rippe women," who have convinced me that I am the luckiest and most loved man in the universe.

To all these individuals and many others who have helped along the way, I am deeply indebted. I hope the final product reflects the dedication and pride as well as the deep caring of all who made it possible. I also hope that this book helps people take the daily actions needed to maintain their general health, rejuvenate their joints, and regain their flexibility, strength, and mobility for a lifetime of active living!

The Joint Health
PRESCRIPTION

Breakthrough Thinking about Joint Problems

The human body contains more than a hundred joints—143, to be exact. Strong, flexible joints are essential for almost every activity of daily living. Whether you are throwing a baseball, lifting a fork, cuddling a grandchild, nodding approval, rising from a chair, or walking from place to place, you depend on your joints. In a sense, healthy joints help make our lives possible.

Unfortunately, however, joint problems are the leading cause of disability in the United States and around the world. Studies show that at any one time, one-third of adults are having problems with at least one joint. Joint inflammation and injuries can cause even simple movements to become painful or impossible, leading to years of misery and an increasingly restricted life.

Up to now, in helping people who have joint problems, there has been a singular emphasis on pain reduction, often primarily through the use of drugs. This approach, although valuable, has tended to mask—rather than treat—the underlying causes of joint pain.

In this book, I present striking new thinking about joint problems. Aging doesn't have to mean pain, increasing restrictions on mobility, or the loss of your ability to lead an active life. As you grow older, you don't have to take more and more medication to relieve joint pain. Instead, by taking the simple steps presented in this book, you can actually rebuild damaged cartilage, rejuvenate your joints, and help your-self to reverse the restrictions on your mobility—and to lead a *more* active life.

Your joints were meant to last a lifetime. Incorporating simple, healthful habits and practices into your daily life, including the break-through plan presented in this book, can help you to prevent joint problems and to regain youthful strength, flexibility, and mobility.

Helping people achieve healthy lifestyles has been the driving passion of my career as a physician. My research laboratory in Shrewsbury, Massachusetts, the Rippe Lifestyle Institute, has become the largest organization studying the impact of lifestyle habits on both short- and long-term health and on the quality of life. At the institute, my colleagues and I have done many studies and helped thousands of people establish healthy programs in the areas of fitness walking, weight management, cholesterol control, and many other health-promoting lifestyle activities. Along the way, I became known as the father of the American walking movement. I am very proud of that distinction.

Thus, when we entered the area of joint health in 1999, it was a natural venture for my laboratory to carry out the first major, strictly controlled scientific study of lifestyle approaches to maintaining and enhancing joint health rather than focusing on medical and pharmaceutical treatment of joint disease.

After planning the study, we put our first small ad in the newspaper, asking people who had mild symptoms of joint discomfort in one or both knees to join us for a landmark study on how to promote healthy joints. Would people care enough about joints—something they rarely think about—to join the study? We weren't sure at first, but the morning the ad appeared, the flood began! We were inundated with phone calls from people who wanted healthy joints.

Within 1 month, several hundred men and women volunteered to take part in our study. Participants came from many different back-grounds and walks of life. They were of all ages and had a variety of symptoms of joint discomfort, ranging from very mild to moderate. We excluded only would-be study participants who already had significant joint disease, because the focus of the study was on preserving joint health rather than on treating joint disease.

Over a 6-month period, we studied more than 200 people. The results were incredible! People who received a gelatin-based dietary supplement achieved significant improvements in a variety of areas, including increased joint strength, flexibility, and mobility along with a number of other helpful benefits, which are detailed in chapter 2.

This study helped us to develop a new paradigm for thinking about joints, which we call the Joint Health Program. The 8-week program that we present in this book is based on innovative concepts that draw on our study and on research into using lifestyle practices to promote both joint health and overall health. Our program focuses on those aspects of daily life—including increased activity, weight management, stretching and strength training, proper nutrition, and, in many instances, supplementation—that will help keep your joints healthy and pain-free throughout your life.

People who have problems with their joints can experience weeks, months, or even years of misery. Joint pain can lead to decreased activity, emotional downs and depression, and diminished quality of life. You can help to avoid those problems or, in some instances, even begin to reverse them. Following the simple plans laid out in this book, you can minimize your risk of joint problems and maximize your joint health—and dramatically improve your quality of life.

New Discoveries to Rejuvenate Your Joints

Understanding Joint Pain

If you think that aching joints affect mostly athletes and older people, think again. Worldwide, an estimated 50 percent of all people over the age of 30 have some problem with at least one joint. Hands and knees lead the problem parade.

- In one study of more than 5,000 people over age 65, almost half of all disability was a direct result of joint problems.
- Another study found that young adults who have had joint injuries are five times more likely to develop osteoarthritis than those who have not had such injuries.
- Each year in the United States, more than 11 million visits to physicians are made for knee problems.
- Since World War II, a number of studies undertaken around the world have found that joint disease contributes to numerous other health conditions, primarily because joint problems prevent people from being physically active. These problems include heart disease, obesity, diabetes, further joint problems, and a poorer quality of life.

Joint problems tend to be what we in medicine call chronic. Although chronic diseases generally do not directly lead to loss of life, they can cause years of misery for those who suffer from them. Your picture of aging may be clouded by fear of being hobbled by arthritis and losing your ability to function independently. But you can do something to change that dismal picture. You can tap the benefits of research to improve your joint health and decrease your likelihood of developing joint problems or to alleviate symptoms if you already have painful joints.

WHAT IS A JOINT, ANYWAY?

Connecting our bones into a movable, versatile, supportive skeletal frame is the task of our joints and the variety of tissues and fluids that comprise their structure.

We have many different kinds of joints, and many are very complex. But all joints (from the ball-and-socket joints of the hips to the hinge joints of the elbows and knees) have a variety of components. These components include the bones that articulate, or connect, at the joint; the cartilage (the soft cushioning between the bones); the various ligaments that attach bone to bone; and the tendons that attach muscle to bone. Problems with any of these structures or the fluid that surrounds them can lead to joint discomfort and decreased function. Conversely, strategies to improve the health of any of these structures can improve the health of the entire joint. For example, two of the amino acids found in gelatin-based supplements—glycine and proline—are essential to rebuilding the cartilage that cushions the joint.

WHAT GOES WRONG WITH JOINTS

When joints are functioning at their best, they enable smooth, pain-free movements of all kinds. These movements may be as delicate as threading a small needle or performing microsurgery or as dynamic as jumping from your car in the rain, opening your umbrella, and sprinting for shelter. Day in and day out, our joints not only perform complex movements large and small but also take the pounding of thousands of pounds of pressure generated in the course of an active, healthy life.

Joints experience a high-stress environment, so it's no wonder that many things can go wrong with them. Repeated trauma to a joint (think of the hands and shoulders of a jackhammer operator or the knees of a carpet layer), for example, can lead to osteoarthritis. Acute injury to a joint (think of a twisted ankle or a sprained wrist) can lead to significant and chronic joint problems. Joints are also susceptible to the effects of infections or diseases of the endocrine glands and to problems with the bones themselves. The stronger and healthier your joints are, the less vulnerable they are to any of these problems.

THE CAUSES OF JOINT PAIN

As you might guess, osteoarthritis is by far the most common joint problem. This form of arthritis results from deterioration of the bone and cartilage, which causes inflammation and, ultimately, pain and dysfunction. Because it causes more than half of all joint problems around the world, I will discuss osteoarthritis throughout this book.

Here is a brief rundown of the various causes of joint pain.

INFLAMMATORY AND DEGENERATIVE CONDITIONS

Inflammation can occur in virtually any part of a joint. In medicine, we call an inflammation an "-itis." Inflammation of the joint is called arthritis, inflammation of the tendon sheath is called tendinitis, and inflammation of the bursae (the flat, fluid-filled sacs that help your joints slide smoothly) is called bursitis.

Arthritis. The term *arthritis* refers to a large family of inflammatory degenerative diseases that includes more than 100 different types of conditions. In all its forms, arthritis is by far the most common joint problem in the United States and the leading cause of disability for people over the age of 65.

The most common form of arthritis is osteoarthritis, a degenerative condition experienced by large numbers of people, usually as they grow older. More than 35 million adults in the United States (one out of seven) have arthritis. Its symptoms include pain, stiffness, and swelling of the joint. As described in chapter 2, the participants in our study of joint health experienced improvements that decreased their likelihood of developing significant osteoarthritis.

Rheumatoid arthritis, which is a type of highly inflammatory arthritis, is the next most common form. It is a systemic disease, meaning that it goes beyond the joints to affect the whole body. It can strike at any age. Other inflammatory types of arthritis include lupus, ankylosing spondylitis, scleroderma, and gout. Rheumatoid arthritis and other forms of inflammatory arthritis are so complex and individual that I will discuss them only in passing.

Bursitis and tendinitis. Bursitis occurs when the fibrous sac (bursa) near a joint becomes inflamed, often as a result of excessive stress or friction. One component of tennis elbow is often bursitis of the elbow. Symptoms include pain (which is made worse by moving the joint), local swelling, and sometimes redness.

Tendinitis is an inflammation of the fibrous sheaths that run outside of tendons. Its symptoms are very similar to those of bursitis.

COMMON JOINT INJURIES

Even if you've never come closer to playing a sport than watching it on TV, you've probably jammed a finger or twisted a knee or ankle at some time. (Maybe you tripped over the dog as you raced from couch to kitchen to get a snack during a timeout.) The most common joint injuries are sprains and dislocations, followed by cartilage injuries.

Sprains. In a sprain, the ligaments that reinforce and support a joint are stretched or torn. Partial tears of ligaments will heal on their own, but if a ligament is completely torn (also called a rupture), it must be repaired surgically. Otherwise, the continuing inflammatory process can severely harm other structures in the joint. A severe rupture can make the joint totally dysfunctional.

Dislocation. A dislocation occurs when bones are forced out of their normal positions in a joint. This often occurs in serious falls and is common in contact sports. The joints of the shoulders, fingers, and thumbs are common sites for this type of injury. When dislocation occurs, it is imperative that the bone ends be returned to their proper position by a physician or other trained medical professional. No matter how successfully an amateur hero handles the procedure in the movies or on TV, in real life an untrained person trying to snap a bone back into its socket usually does more harm than good.

Cartilage injuries. Torn cartilage in the knee is among the most common injuries of this type, particularly in those who play contact sports or sports that require sudden twisting motions, such as tennis or basketball. It may seem that these injuries affect mostly elite athletes, but recreational players also regularly experience them. You can even tear cartilage by lunging to catch Grandma's heirloom vase that the baby just knocked off the table. These injuries often require surgery to remove fragments of torn cartilage so that they don't cause significant inflammation of the joint. When the tear in the cartilage is relatively minor, physical therapy may be recommended to strengthen the muscles around the affected joint (typically the knee).

ARE YOU AT RISK FOR JOINT PROBLEMS?

Over the past 50 years, we've learned a great deal about who's most likely to develop joint problems. Although there is a wide variety of contributing factors, seven leading risk characteristics have been identified. The good news is that if you understand these factors, you can take steps to diminish your own risk.

AGE

Joint problems increase with age. That's a sad fact of life. But even though you can't do anything about your chronological age, you can do a great deal about your "physiological" age—the age that reflects how well you have taken care of your body. The older you are, the more important it is that you adopt a strategy for improving and protecting your joint health.

FEMALE GENDER

For reasons that are poorly understood, women tend to have more joint problems than men do. This is especially true after menopause. For this reason, women should pay particular attention to the factors that have been identified for improving joint health.

WEIGHT

Being overweight or obese can significantly increase your risk of joint problems in general and osteoarthritis in particular. In fact, obesity is the leading cause of osteoarthritis in women and the second leading cause (behind prior injuries) in men. Extra pounds place extra stress on the joints that must support that weight, especially the knees and hips. This stress can also push joints out of proper alignment, further injuring them. For these reasons, weight management is an important part of maintaining joint health.

PREVIOUS INJURY

People often come to me complaining of aching joints that have bothered them for many years. Frequently, the initial events that caused the long-term joint problems were athletic or other types of injuries. Although injuries cannot be totally prevented, keeping your muscles strong for daily living and conditioning your body for specific sports and recreational activities can go a long way toward decreasing the likelihood of joint injury and subsequent problems.

OCCUPATIONAL HISTORY

Various studies have shown that people in occupations that require repetitive squatting or kneeling have an increased likelihood of problems in the joints that are put under the most stress. Although most people cannot change their occupations, adopting certain preventive measures can reduce this risk. In addition, people who engage in active leisure pursuits that use repetitive motions (such as gardening or weekend tennis) should pay particular attention to joint health to minimize the likelihood of injury or other problems.

MUSCLE WEAKNESS

As people grow older, their muscles typically become weaker. There is a complex interplay between muscle and joint, and muscle weakness often leads to a joint problem rather than a joint problem leading to muscle weakness. Stretching and strength-building exercises, such as those presented in chapter 7, are excellent ways to keep your muscles, particularly those around vulnerable joints, strong for life. Research has shown that even people in their eighties and nineties can gain function and mobility using such exercises.

BONE PROBLEMS

Various bone diseases (including osteoporosis) and bone injuries can lead to joint problems. Throughout this book, I will discuss ways to keep your bones healthy for life.

SIGNS AND SYMPTOMS OF UNHEALTHY JOINTS

In medicine, we make a distinction between symptoms, which are what a patient experiences, and signs, which are what a doctor typically discovers.

Anyone who has had problems with a joint knows the main symptoms, starting with pain. Such pain may be worse either at rest or during activity. Other common symptoms include morning joint stiffness, buckling or instability, and diminished function (such as range of motion) of the joint.

The signs of problems that a physician may notice include enlargement of the bones around the joint, tenderness when the joint is touched, heat or extra fluid in the joint, limited range of motion, or deformity. All of these signs can be evaluated by a trained physician. If you have any of these indicators of joint problems, you should consult your physician before undertaking the 8-Week Joint Health Program described in the following chapters. (See chapter 12 for more information about medical evaluation of joint problems.)

ENDING AND PREVENTING JOINT PAIN

Our joints rely on complex, durable structures to perform the wonderfully varied motions of our daily lives. You can end or prevent joint pain by keeping these complex mechanisms healthy and functioning smoothly. In the rest of this book, I'll show you the simple lifestyle steps that you can take to end joint pain, preserve or regain your flexibility, and keep your joints healthy for a lifetime.

The first step is "use it or lose it!" It's a fairly common misconception that people who walk or run regularly for exercise are susceptible to developing joint problems. Although a lifetime of physical activity is no guarantee that you will avoid joint problems, numerous studies have shown that people who are involved in healthful activities such as walking or running significantly decrease their likelihood of developing joint problems. In one major study, less than 2 percent of people who classified themselves as regular walkers or runners experienced significant joint problems later in their lives. Properly chosen and structured physical activity can also help treat existing joint problems.

The next step is to keep your muscles strong. People who maintain strong muscles seem to have fewer joint problems than those who allow their muscles to grow weak. For this reason, following a program that involves regular walking or running as well as strength training is one of the best means of promoting joint health. Strength training also plays a big role in recovering joint health and function.

Eating healthfully is the third "must" for promoting joint health. Proper nutrition, including supplementation when appropriate, can help ensure that your body gets the building blocks it needs to create and maintain healthy tissues and bones. Proper nutrition is also essential for weight management.

HOW THIS BOOK AND THE 8-WEEK JOINT HEALTH PROGRAM CAN HELP

The Joint Health Prescription provides an 8-week action plan to help you reach two major goals:

1. To manage the pain and other symptoms of joint problems if they already exist
2. To keep joints healthy for a lifetime of active living

The 8-Week Joint Health Program begins with simple tests, grouped in an easy-to-use format, that enable you to determine your current level of joint health and have a benchmark to use as it improves.

Then, I provide specific, appropriate action plans to improve your joint health. Many of these involve simple daily activities, such as regular exercise, proper nutrition, strength training, and stretching, as well as weight management. I also recommend supplementation in many instances. Like many of the subjects in our study, you may benefit from taking a gelatin-based supplement. I discuss who can achieve the most benefit from taking such a supplement and how to integrate it into your life. I also provide guidance about the bewildering array of supplements and medicines that are available to treat joint problems.

Because health challenges change as we grow older, I provide specific advice for different age groups. I share tips about how to talk to your physician about joint health before you develop problems or about the most modern techniques for treating problems if you already have pain.

I tell the inspiring stories of individuals, including some who participated in our study, who are trying to improve their joint health so that they can gain all the physical and mental health benefits of an active lifestyle. You will find many of your challenges, goals, and achievements mirrored in their experiences.

Simple steps that you can take in your daily life can go a long way toward keeping your joints healthy for a lifetime. That is what *The Joint Health Prescription* is all about—giving you a plan for joint health that will help you achieve the quality of life you want and deserve.

A Landmark Study on Joint Health

What keeps joints healthy? Research has shown that many risk factors for joint disease have to do with daily lifestyle decisions and habits. We know, for example, that people who maintain proper body weight and keep their muscles strong are less likely to experience joint problems than those who are overweight or allow their muscles to become weak. People who exercise regularly, even if they have osteoarthritis, have less functional decline and less joint pain than people who don't exercise regularly.

On the basis of existing scientific evidence about the possible role of certain nutritional substances in promoting joint health, my research institute designed a scientifically rigorous study to assess the effectiveness of supplementation with gelatin fortified with vitamin C and calcium (our study used Knox NutraJoint). We proposed a large study (more than 200 participants) using a randomized, prospective, double-blind, placebo-controlled trial to determine whether the gelatin-based supplement helped to improve participants' scores on various indexes of joint health by decreasing pain and stiffness and improving mobility and function, for example.

Let's look for a minute at the factors that make this kind of study so rigorous and consequently make the information that's produced so valuable.

- In a *randomized* study, the people who volunteer for the study are randomly assigned to either a group that receives the active ingredient being tested or a group that receives a placebo, a substance that looks exactly like the test substance but does not contain the active ingredient.
- *Prospective* means that the study looks forward rather than backward in time. In other words, it follows both groups of participants to determine what happens to them over the period of the study rather than starting with participants with given outcomes and then looking back to determine what may have caused those outcomes.
- In a *double-blind* study, neither the researchers nor the subjects know which subjects are receiving active substances and which the placebos. This means that the people who randomize the groups don't carry out the actual testing and research.
- *Placebo-controlled* means that all participants get substances that look exactly alike (and taste alike, if applicable) so they cannot know whether they have the test product or the placebo. In our study, everyone got a powder.

This very strong type of scientific study, which is used throughout the pharmaceutical industry to test new drug products, is designed to eliminate any potential bias on the part of either the subjects or the investigators.

DEVELOPING THE STUDY

After selecting a design, the study developers looked at what needed to be tested, the best researchers to conduct the testing, and the most appropriate subjects for the test.

THE TEST SUPPLEMENT

The food scientists were not simply guessing when they designed the supplement that was tested. Earlier evidence suggested that each of the ingredients used in the supplement could individually benefit components of joints.

- Gelatin is high in two amino acids, proline and glycine, that are critical to building and repairing the cartilage in joints. Because cartilage has a relatively poor blood supply, it is often difficult for these amino acids to be transported through the bloodstream so that repair of this vital structure in the joint can occur. The premise for the study was the theory that consuming gelatin can increase the amount of proline and glycine available to the joints as building blocks to keep cartilage in good repair.

◾ Vitamin C was added to the supplement because of data from the Framingham Osteoarthritis Study, which showed that people who consumed higher levels of vitamin C on a regular basis had a decreased incidence of arthritis of the joints.

◾ Calcium was included because it is vital to bone health and repair.

THE RESEARCHERS

A team of scientists was assembled to develop and supervise the study at the Rippe Lifestyle Institute in Shrewsbury, Massachusetts. This team included a well-known rheumatologist, Eric Jacobson, M.D. (rheumatology is the study of joint disease and joint health), and a well-known biomechanist, Mark Rowinski, Ph.D. (biomechanics is the study of the motion of the joints), as well as other physicians, exercise physiologists, and nurses. Each investigator contributed a particular expertise to the study.

THE TESTS

Our team of researchers put together the following series of tests to provide a very comprehensive set of investigations in the area of joint health.

◾ A 6-minute walking test, which measured how far participants could walk in 6 minutes; it is a good test of the functional capacity of the knee and hip.

◾ A 50-foot walking test, which determined how fast participants could walk a distance of 50 feet; it is a good measurement of mobility.

◾ A pain, stiffness, and mobility questionnaire, which asked participants to evaluate how much pain they experienced when walking, climbing a flight of stairs, and doing other activities of daily living; it was used to assess the levels of pain, stiffness, and mobility in the knee joint.

- A quality of life questionnaire, which determined the impact of knee discomfort on the participants' lives.
- Range of motion assessments, which determined the level of flexibility in the knee joint.
- Isokinetic and isometric leg strength assessments, which used sophisticated, high-tech instrumentation to provide the most objective evidence of the strength and functional ability of the knee.

THE SUBJECTS

The first criterion for recruiting subjects for the study was that they belong to the population most affected by joint problems—people between the ages of 40 and 85. In addition, they had to have knee pain in at least one knee, morning stiffness in the knee lasting less than 30 minutes, and several findings on physical examination by a researcher, such as bony tenderness and bony enlargement. People who met all of these criteria were eligible for the study.

In addition, the subjects had to be willing to maintain stable body weights throughout the study, and, if they were taking medications for their knee pain, they had to be willing to maintain stable doses of these medications and keep diaries documenting their daily intakes.

People could not participate if they had any known rheumatologic disease other than these symptoms of possible mild osteoarthritis or if they had any significant health problem that would prohibit them from participating in the intense procedures of the study.

THE PROTOCOL

Those who qualified for the study and were willing to participate had to agree to come to the research center 18 times over a 14-week period and undergo a series of tests designed to assess virtually every aspect of joint health. The study required a real commitment from participants to help advance science in this important area.

LAUNCHING THE STUDY

Many people were eager to participate. The first small ad drew more than 75 responses in 2 days. Respondents to additional ads filled all available testing slots at our laboratory. Over the 6 months that we recruited subjects, 567 people volunteered. Out of the number who expressed interest, 250 were eventually accepted into the trial, and nearly 200 of them completed the 14-week protocol.

The individuals who participated in the study were very representative of people with mild knee pain. Approximately half were men and half were women, with an average age of 57. They came from all walks of life. For example:

- Marge and Al Lucier, both in their seventies, are retirees who wanted to get around more freely.
- Ron Heirtzler, 60, is a carpenter who's up and down all day, putting stress on his knees; pain was part of the job.
- Susan Caron, 42, who runs her own cleaning service for residences and offices, spends a lot of time on troubled knees. Her doctor predicted early knee replacement.

HOW THE STUDY WAS DONE

During the study period, participants were asked to consume one scoop (10 grams) of the powder they had received (either the fortified gelatin-based supplement or a placebo) each morning in orange juice or coffee. During this period, they also had to visit the laboratory 18 times for various tests. Overall, the study took 6 months because laboratory testing required staggered starts to accommodate so many participants.

Compliance with this tough regimen was very high. In fact, the participants consumed more than 92 percent of all of the supplement or placebo that they were asked to use. They did not mind taking the supplement every day, which is important because taking it daily gives the most dramatic benefits.

THE RESULTS

At the end of the study, the investigators and subjects were allowed to see who had been taking the supplements and who had been on the placebos. The study findings were very encouraging for those of us working for healthy joints.

Both the participants who received the gelatin supplement and those who received the placebos showed marked improvements on the 6-minute walk and the 50-foot walk; on their pain, stiffness, and mobility scores; and in their quality of life, including decreases in body pain and increases in healthy functioning.

In the areas of isokinetic and isometric strength, however, which provide the most objective assessment of joint health, the supplement demonstrated clear superiority to the placebo. These tests, which put joints under maximum stress, showed that the supplement was significantly more effective than the placebo in virtually every parameter tested. Furthermore, when people who had moderate joint pain were evaluated separately from those who had very mild pain, the supplement outperformed the placebo even more significantly in those with moderate pain.

IMPLICATIONS OF THE FINDINGS

The study participants who took the gelatin-based supplement trended toward more improvement in tests of function, such as the walking tests; more decreases in symptoms of pain and stiffness; and more improvements in mobility and quality of life than participants who received the placebo. In addition, the high-tech assessments of joint health showed significantly more benefits from the supplement than from the placebo. The results of those tests imply that it is not just coincidence that participants who received the gelatin-based supplement trended toward greater improvement on the other measurements, and they indicate the possibility that over a longer period than 14 weeks, the trend could become statistically significant.

The implications of these findings are enormous. We now have objective evidence that by taking something as simple as a supplement combining gelatin, vitamin C, and calcium, people can achieve significant improvements in measurements of joint health. If you already have joint problems, this is a simple way to decrease the likelihood that you will develop more significant problems. If you have no joint problems, this practice could potentially increase your likelihood of maintaining healthy joints into the future. Further studies are needed to determine whether people who have severe joint problems can also benefit from such a regimen.

In *The Joint Health Prescription*, I have put the objective findings of this study into a total program that shows you how to use a variety of scientifically validated practices and habits to keep your joints healthy for a lifetime of active living.

How did our sample participants fare?

Marge Lucier, who was in the group that received the supplement, has found that she has an easier time walking up stairs and on hilly land. Her husband, Al, was in the placebo group. After the study, he began to take the gelatin-based supplement that was tested.

Ron Heirtzler, the carpenter, was in the group taking the supplement, and he has continued to use it. He won't miss a day, he says, because it makes a difference that he can feel.

Susan Caron says that as she goes about her cleaning business now, she notices that her knees rebound more quickly after a hard day's work. She continues to take the supplement regularly.

Many other participants told us similar stories of the benefits they achieved. Following the simple plans in this book, you may enjoy the same positive results.

The Program to Heal and Protect Your Joints

Getting Started with the 8-Week Joint Health Program

Your situation may resemble that of Mary Brown, a participant in our research study on joint health. Mary called to ask about joining the study because her knees were bothering her. The trouble began after she started doing a step aerobics program that she had seen on television. Her knees hurt most when she went up and down stairs.

Mary was worried. Her grandmother had been obese and had to have both knees replaced. Her father, who was also overweight, had bad knees that made it very difficult for him to move about. She wanted to avoid a similar future.

When Mary entered the study, she feared that she had been randomly assigned to the placebo group because she did not notice any change for the first few weeks (aren't we all impatient?). After 4 to 6 weeks, however, she began to notice a real improvement in her knee function. This gradual but significant improvement continued throughout the remainder of the study. By the end of that time, Mary was feeling great.

Mary continues to take a gelatin-based supplement daily. She is now able to enjoy all of the pleasurable activities of being an active grandmother and frequently baby-sits for her two preschool-age grandchildren. She also was thrilled that she was able to participate in an 18-mile, 2-day walk.

Mary's experience illustrates a number of important points about joint health. First, it is important not to rush into an exercise program, even the activity components of my 8-Week Joint Health Program, particularly if you have previously been sedentary. On the basis of a television program, Mary chose aerobic stepping, an activity that's particularly stressful to the knees, and she experienced the painful result of that stress. Before beginning my program, read through all the elements, understand them, take the simple tests in chapter 4, and adapt the program to fit your condition and needs.

Second, you need to take the steps that are right for your physical condition and goals. As Mary participated in the study and took the gelatin-based supplement, she gradually experienced an improvement in knee function. She also began to walk regularly, an activity that contributes to joint health and helps maintain weight, which will also help her achieve pain-free joints.

Third, the improvement in Mary's joint health enhanced her quality of life because she was able to do the things she wanted with ease and enjoyment. Other participants in the study had similar results.

WHAT THE PROGRAM WILL DO FOR YOU

If you are already experiencing some problems with your joints, following the simple regimen of the Joint Health Program can begin to improve your joint function in just 8 weeks. If your joints are not troublesome, the program will help keep them healthy and decrease your risk of ever having joint pain, dysfunction, or other problems.

The great thing about the recommendations in the 8-Week Joint Health Program is that they are good for everybody! They are also good for your whole body, not just your joints. We know, for example, that active people cut their risk of heart disease in half and that both activity and proper nutrition are very important for weight management. If you follow the simple plans outlined for each element of the program, you will find that you feel better, more in control, and happier about your life than ever before.

Let's start with a brief overview of the program. Chapters 4 through 10 provide step-by-step instructions and recommendations to help you accomplish each element of your 8-week program, from physical activity to nutrition. Chapter 11 shows you how to maintain what you've accomplished for a lifetime. Here's a brief summary of each chapter's objective and contents.

CHAPTER 4: TESTING THE HEALTH OF YOUR JOINTS

Your program begins with a few simple tests that you can take to determine the current health of your joints. It is important to establish this baseline assessment so that you can customize the program to fit your needs and also measure how much your joints improve, particularly if you are currently having problems. Some of the tests are pencil-and-paper tests; others require that you perform simple activities such as walking or stretching. You can do them all in 2 hours or less. To do the walk tests, you will need a good pair of walking shoes, loose clothing appropriate for walking, and a stopwatch.

CHAPTER 5: WALKING

When I was in medical school 25 years ago, many people who engaged in vigorous walking programs—and certainly those who already had joint problems—were told that they should take it easy. How times have changed! Thanks to extensive research, we now know that regular physical activity, such as walking, can be one of the best things you can do to maintain and improve joint health. This chapter highlights the reasons that walking benefits joints. It also summarizes the pros and cons of other forms of exercise and shows you how to take special precautions for activities that may put extra stress on your joints. There is also a graduated series of 8-week walking programs that are designed to help improve joint health and can also be adapted for other activities, such as bicycling or swimming.

CHAPTER 6: GETTING MORE ACTIVITY EVERY DAY

Here, I show you how common activities such as gardening, mowing, and sweeping can help maintain healthy joints, and I offer ways to reduce any risk to your joints from these activities. The modern understanding of physical activity and health is that people who are physically active significantly lower their risks for various chronic diseases. By remaining active, you may not only improve your joint health but also live a healthier, happier life.

CHAPTER 7: STRETCHING AND STRENGTHENING

Flexibility and muscle tone are important for joint health. Stretching and strength-training programs can improve these and other factors that affect your joints. In addition to improving flexibility, stretching programs help increase mobility and function. Strength training can be of benefit both to people with no joint problems and to those who have arthritis. You'll learn stretches that target various joints as well as how to determine which strength-training program is right for you; how to select a strength-training facility, if desired; and how to perform simple strength-training exercises at home. There is also a graduated series of 8-week programs designed to optimize muscle strength around your joints.

CHAPTER 8: MANAGING YOUR WEIGHT

Because being overweight or obese is clearly associated with an increased risk of joint problems, weight management is highly effective for improving and maintaining joint health and treating joint injury. Many people, however, tend to overlook its importance. This chapter outlines the proper steps for weight management and provides simple guidance on ways to manage your weight as a means of improving your joint health.

CHAPTER 9: EATING FOR JOINT HEALTH

Good information about nutrition can be very helpful in controlling your weight, reducing your risk of chronic disease, and improving your joint health. Unfortunately, a tremendous amount of misinformation is always circulating about foods that may either help or hurt joint health. This chapter cuts through the hype and the hoopla to provide the best available advice, based on scientific findings, on using nutrition and healthful eating to enhance joint health.

CHAPTER 10: USING SUPPLEMENTS WISELY

The marketplace is filled with a bewildering variety of supplements that have been touted either as cures for arthritis or as adjuncts to joint health. This chapter examines all the available supplements, including hydrolyzed gelatin-based supplements, glucosamine, chondroitin, and shark cartilage, and provides objective evidence about any claims about the supplements' benefit to joints. You'll learn what the scientific evidence shows for and against each supplement—what is proven and not proven—and get some guidance about choices to meet your personal needs.

CHAPTER 11: MAINTAINING HEALTHY JOINTS FOR LIFE

After 8 weeks of participation in the research study, many of the subjects trended toward improvement in their overall joint health. After 14 weeks, the improvements were clearly established. The goal, of course, is to maintain joint health for a lifetime, so chapter 11 presents suggestions for using the practices that you learn in the first 8-week programs as ongoing strategies to ensure that your joints stay healthy.

As you will see, the lifestyle recommendations and specific regimens in this program can help decrease or end any existing joint pain that you may have, significantly reduce your risk of developing joint problems, and greatly improve your quality of life. In just 8 weeks, you can be on track for a lifetime of healthy, pain-free, functional joints.

Testing the Health of Your Joints

As the king said in *Alice's Adventures in Wonderland*, let's begin at the beginning. When it comes to joint health, the beginning is testing your joints to find out their current state of health. With the easy tests that follow, which you can do in about 2 hours max, you can find out what you need to know about your joints in order to get started on the 8-Week Joint Health Program.

A word of caution: Don't skip the tests. Many people say, "Well, I'll just do the programs and take the tests later, when my joints are in better shape." If you do that, you won't know the right level at which to start your program based on your current joint health or have a concrete baseline against which to judge your progress. Both of these factors are important to success, so make the time and take the tests.

The tests will help you assess the major aspects of joint health and several related factors. Record your scores on the Joint Health Profile Card on page 55, and use your findings to help customize the program to fit your needs. Here's a summary of what you'll be testing.

Symptoms. Of course, you need to be aware of any symptoms you have that may be linked to your joints. Many people ignore their joints, even shrugging off a twinge or two, until more major problems occur. Filling out the questionnaire will help you look at any symptoms you may have and give you a sense of their significance.

Function. You'll take two simple tests that were used by the subjects in my study—the 6-minute walk and the 50-foot walk. They will help you assess how well your knees and hips function as well as give you a sense of the health of the joints connecting the vertebrae in your back. Because we use our hands in almost everything we do, I've added a simple hand-stretch test for your finger and wrist joints.

Flexibility and strength. Flexibility and muscle strength are both related to joint health. The sit-and-reach test assesses the flexibility of your lower back, hips, and legs. The leg-extension test helps you gauge lower-body strength.

Impact of joint health on quality of life. We all want to improve our quality of life. This questionnaire helps you judge to what extent joint problems may be affecting your emotional and physical well-being.

Other tests. Factors such as being sedentary or overweight, which affect your joint health, also affect the level at which you should begin your program. The physical activity questionnaire and the body mass index assessment will help you get a handle on these factors.

PREPARING TO TAKE THE TESTS

Taking a moment to assemble the items you need for the tests will make your test time easier, shorter, and more fun. Here's the list.

- A pair of good walking shoes
- Loose, comfortable clothing
- A tape measure to measure distances for the 50-foot walk and 6-minute walk
- A stopwatch to time yourself on the 50-foot walk and 6-minute walk (and, if you're not shy, a friend to cheer you along and time you)
- A sharpened pencil to record your answers on the questionnaires
- A yardstick and masking tape for the sit-and-reach test
- A 10-pound ankle weight (or two 5-pound weights) for the leg-extension test
- A sturdy, straight-backed chair

It's also a good idea to find a measured track, since you will need to record how far you walk in the 6-minute walk. Most high schools and colleges have tracks, as do many health clubs and YMCAs. As a last resort, you can use a tape measure to mark out 150 or 75 feet (50 or 25 yards) on a flat sidewalk or driveway and walk back and forth on it.

Finally, read through all the instructions before beginning the tests.

THE JOINT HEALTH INDEX

This simple pencil-and-paper test determines how much discomfort or decreased function you have when it comes to walking and performing the activities of daily living. The test will also ask you to evaluate how much pain you have when performing certain activities in your daily life.

HIPS AND KNEES

For each section, use the number scale to answer the questions, then add the numbers to find your total for that section.

Part A: Frequency of Pain

4	3	2	1	0
Always	Almost Always	Sometimes	Almost Never	Never

1. When you are lying in bed at night, do you experience any joint pain in your hips or knees?

2. Do you experience any joint pain in your hips or knees when walking up or down a flight of stairs?

3. When getting up from a sitting position *without* the help of your arms, do you experience any joint pain in your hips or knees?

4. Do you experience any joint pain in your hips or knees when you walk 300 feet?

Score for Part A

Part B: Severity of Pain

4	3	2	1	0
Agonizing Pain	Severe Pain	Moderate Pain	Slight Pain	No Pain

1. When you are lying in bed at night, do you experience any joint pain in your hips or knees?

2. Do you experience any joint pain in your hips or knees when walking up or down a flight of stairs?

3. When getting up from a sitting position *without* the help of your arms, do you experience any joint pain in your hips or knees?

4. Do you experience any joint pain in your hips or knees when you walk 300 feet?

Score for Part B

Part C: Duration of Stiffness

4	3	2	1	0
30+ min	16–30 min	6–15 min	1–5 min	No Stiffness

1. When you wake up in the morning, do you experience any joint stiffness in your hips or knees?

(*Note*: If you score a 4 on this question, please see your doctor; your joint problem may not be primarily osteoarthritis.)

Score for Part C

Total Score

Part A

Part B

Part C

TOTAL

Check your total score against the key below to find your level for the walking and lower-body strength programs.

35–22	21–8	7–0
Level 1	**Level 2**	**Level 3**

FINGERS

For each section, use the number scale to answer the questions, then add the numbers to find your total for that section.

Part A: Frequency of Pain

4	3	2	1	0
Always	Almost Always	Sometimes	Almost Never	Never

1. When pulling open a door, do you experience any joint pain in your fingers?

2. Do you experience any joint pain in your fingers when writing a short note?

3. Do you experience any joint pain in your fingers when you drive?

4. When you are lying in bed at night, do you experience any joint pain in your fingers?

Score for Part A

Part B: Severity of Pain

4	3	2	1	0
Agonizing Pain	Severe Pain	Moderate Pain	Slight Pain	No Pain

1. When pulling open a door, do you experience any joint pain in your fingers?

2. Do you experience any joint pain in your fingers when writing a short note?

3. Do you experience any joint pain in your fingers when you drive?

4. When you are lying in bed at night, do you experience any joint pain in your fingers? ☐

Score for Part B ▨

Part C: Duration of Stiffness

4	3	2	1	0
30+ min	16–30 min	6–15 min	1–5 min	No Stiffness

1. When you wake up in the morning, do you experience any joint stiffness in your fingers? ☐

(*Note:* If you score a 4 on this question, please see your doctor; your joint problem may not be primarily osteoarthritis.)

Score for Part C ▨

Total Score

Part A	☐
Part B	☐
Part C	☐
TOTAL	▨

Check your total score against the key below to find your level for the dexterity program.

35–22	21–8	7–0
Level 1	**Level 2**	**Level 3**

BACK AND NECK

For each section, use the number scale to answer the questions, then add the numbers to find your total for that section.

Part A: Frequency of Pain

4	3	2	1	0
Always	Almost Always	Sometimes	Almost Never	Never

1. When you are lying in bed at night, do you experience any joint pain in your back or neck?

2. When seated for a short time (less than 30 minutes), do you experience any joint pain in your back or neck?

3. Do you experience any joint pain in your back or neck when you walk 300 feet?

Score for Part A

Part B: Severity of Pain

4	3	2	1	0
Agonizing Pain	Severe Pain	Moderate Pain	Slight Pain	No Pain

1. When you are lying in bed at night, do you experience any joint pain in your back or neck?

2. When seated for a short time (less than 30 minutes), do you experience any joint pain in your back or neck?

3. Do you experience any joint pain in your back or neck when you walk 300 feet?

Score for Part B

Part C: Duration of Stiffness

4	3	2	1	0
30+ min	16–30 min	6–15 min	1–5 min	No Stiffness

1. When you wake up in the morning, do you experience any joint stiffness in your back or neck?

   (*Note*: If you score a 4 on this question, please see your doctor; your joint problem may not be primarily osteoarthritis.)

Score for Part C

Total Score

Part A

Part B

Part C

TOTAL

Check your total score against the key below to find your level for the upper-body strength program.

35–22	21–8	7–0
Level 1	Level 2	Level 3

FUNCTIONAL JOINT HEALTH TESTS

These tests gauge how much functional difficulty you have with your hips or knees when you walk. The first test, the 6-minute walk, is designed to determine the overall function of your knees and hips. The second test, the 50-foot walk, is designed to determine your level of mobility.

It may be a good idea to take a yardstick and masking tape along to your walking test site so you can do the sit-and-reach flexibility test after finishing the walking tests, while your muscles are warm and loose.

THE 6-MINUTE WALK TEST

This is a simple yet strongly validated test that measures both mobility and general fitness. You need a measured area (preferably an athletic track), good walking shoes, a stopwatch, a tape measure, and two objects (such as coins) to mark the spots where you start and stop walking.

1. Warm up by walking slowly for 4 to 5 minutes, gradually increasing your pace. Do some light stretches (the Level 1 stretching program in chapter 7 is fine).
2. Stand at your starting mark, then simultaneously start your stopwatch and begin walking. Keep walking until the stopwatch hits 6 minutes. (If you are walking laps on a short, measured distance, keep track of the number of laps as you go. Here's where a helper could be especially handy.)
3. When you have walked for 6 minutes, stop and mark the spot where you stopped, then measure or estimate the distance from there back to the starting point. Add that distance to the total from your completed laps or premeasured course.
4. Record that total distance on your Joint Health Profile Card on page 55.
5. To determine what level of function your test results indicate, compare your results with the marks for your age and gender in the following chart, then note that level on your profile card.

6-MINUTE WALK RATINGS

		AGE					
		30–39	40–49	50–59	60–69	70–79	80+
	LEVEL	DISTANCE (ft)					
MEN	1	<1,600	<1,500	<1,400	<1,300	<1,200	<1,100
	2	1,600–2,300	1,500–2,200	1,400–2,000	1,300–1,900	1,200–1,800	1,100–1,700
	3	>2,300	>2,200	>2,000	>1,900	>1,800	>1,700
WOMEN	1	<1,500	<1,400	<1,300	<1,200	<1,100	<1,000
	2	1,500–2,200	1,400–2,100	1,300–1,900	1,200–1,800	1,100–1,700	1,000–1,600
	3	>2,200	>2,100	>1,900	>1,800	>1,700	>1,600

< = less than; > = more than

THE 50-FOOT WALK TEST

To take this test, you'll need a stopwatch that is accurate to tenths of a second and a straight line 50 feet long, measured on a flat surface. You may time yourself or have someone else do it.

1. If you are not warmed up from the 6-minute walk, walk slowly for 4 to 5 minutes, gradually increasing your pace. Do some light stretches, such as those for Level 1 in chapter 7.
2. Start at the beginning of the 50-foot line you measured. Simultaneously start the stopwatch and begin to walk the 50 feet as fast as you can without jogging. Stop timing as you cross the end mark.
3. Record your time in seconds to the closest tenth of a second on your Joint Health Profile Card.
4. To determine what level of function your test results indicate, compare your results with the marks for your age and gender in the chart on page 42 and record that level on your profile card.

50-FOOT WALK RATINGS

	LEVEL	\multicolumn{6}{c}{AGE}

	LEVEL	30–39	40–49	50–59	60–69	70–79	80+
		\multicolumn{6}{c}{TIME (sec)}
MEN	1	>11.2	>11.9	>12.8	>13.8	>15.0	>16.3
	2	11.2–7.9	11.9–8.2	12.8–9.1	13.8–9.5	15.0–9.9	16.3–10.6
	3	<7.9	<8.2	<9.1	<9.5	<9.9	<10.6
WOMEN	1	>11.9	>12.8	>13.8	>15.0	>16.3	>17.9
	2	11.9–8.2	12.8–9.1	13.8–9.5	15.0–9.9	16.3–10.6	17.9–11.2
	3	<8.2	<9.1	<9.5	<9.9	<10.6	<11.2

< = less than; > = more than

THE HAND-STRETCH TEST

This test assesses the level of function in your fingers. Although fingers are not usually singled out for individual exercise, you need to exercise them because they are the joints most commonly affected by osteoarthritis.

For this test, you will need a stopwatch or a watch with a sweep second hand.

1. Sit in front of a table or other flat surface, make a fist with one hand, and rest it on the table so that the heel of your hand is flat on the table.
2. Prepare to time yourself for 30 seconds.
3. Extend your hand so that your palm and fingers are flat on the table, then bring your hand back into a fist.
4. Continue to quickly stretch and retract your hand for 30 seconds, counting the repetitions as you go.
5. Repeat the exercise with the other hand.
6. Record either the lower number of repetitions that you were able to do or an average of the scores for both hands on the Joint Health Profile Card.

HAND-STRETCH RATINGS

		AGE					
		30–39	40–49	50–59	60–69	70–79	80+
	LEVEL	REPETITIONS (30 sec)					
MEN AND WOMEN	1	<30	<28	<25	<22	<19	<16
	2	30–40	28–38	25–35	22–32	19–29	16–26
	3	>40	>38	>35	>32	>29	>26

< = less than; > = more than

7. To determine what level of function your test results indicate, compare them with the marks for your age in the chart above and record that level on your profile card.

THE SIT-AND-REACH TEST

This test is easy to perform. Although it specifically assesses the flexibility of your lower back, hips, and legs, it also provides a good estimate of your overall flexibility. First, place a yardstick on the floor (or other level surface such as a sidewalk, driveway, or track), then put a piece of masking tape on the floor on both sides of the yardstick, horizontally and even with the 15-inch mark.

1. If you are not warmed up from taking the walk tests, warm up with slow walking and light stretching.
2. Sit with your legs straight on either side of the yardstick (with the 1-inch end closest to you) and your heels about 12 inches apart. Position yourself so that your heels touch the edges of the masking tape.
3. Stretch out your arms, reach forward as far as possible, and touch the yardstick, noting the inch mark nearest to where you touch. *Caution:* Do not force your "reach." If you feel pain in your legs, knees, or back, stop at that point. Do the test with slow, controlled movements; rapid or jerky movements could result in a pulled muscle.

SIT-AND-REACH RATINGS

	LEVEL	30–39	40–49	50–59	60–69	70–79	80+
		AGE					
		REACH (in)					
MEN	1	<8	<7	<6	<5	<4	<3
MEN	2	8–10	7–9	6–8	5–7	4–6	3–5
MEN	3	>10	>9	>8	>7	>6	>5
WOMEN	1	<11	<10	<9	<8	<7	<6
WOMEN	2	11–13	10–12	9–11	8–10	7–9	6–8
WOMEN	3	>13	>12	>11	>10	>9	>8

<=less than; >=more than

4. Do the test three times and record the longest reach on your Joint Health Profile Card.
5. Compare your results with those for your age and gender in the chart above to determine the appropriate level for your stretching program, then record the level on your profile card.

THE LEG-EXTENSION STRENGTH TEST

For this test, you perform leg extensions with a 10-pound weight (or two 5-pound weights) attached to your ankle. You will also need a stopwatch or a watch with a sweep second hand and a sturdy, straight-backed chair to sit on.

1. Warm up with light stretching.
2. Sit on the chair with your knees bent at a 90-degree angle, with a weight on one ankle and your feet just barely touching the floor.
3. Prepare to time yourself for 10 seconds.
4. Extend the weighted leg straight out, parallel to the floor, then lower it until your foot is resting lightly on the floor again. Count the number of completed leg extensions you can do in 10 seconds.

As you perform the exercise, be careful not to lock your knee in the horizontal position, and avoid bouncing your heel off the floor; your goal is to use quick but controlled movements. To achieve accurate results, it is essential to swing the weighted leg through the full range of motion from vertical to horizontal on each repetition. Do not overexert yourself, and don't hold your breath during the exercise. Exhale each time you extend your leg. Stop if you have any sharp pain.

5. When you complete the test with one leg, rest for 2 minutes, then switch the weight to the other ankle and repeat.

6. On your Joint Health Profile Card, record the lower number of extensions that you were able to perform or an average of the scores for both legs. If you aren't able to complete any full extensions due to your joint discomfort, just do the best you can. Remember that these are your baseline measurements, and your strength will improve by the end of the 8-week program.

7. To determine what level of function your test results indicate, compare them with the marks for your age and gender in the chart below and record that level on your profile card.

LEG-EXTENSION RATINGS

		AGE					
		30–39	40–49	50–59	60–69	70–79	80+
	LEVEL	REPETITIONS (10 sec)					
MEN	1	<6	<6	<5	<4	<3	<3
	2	6–8	6–8	5–8	4–7	3–7	3–7
	3	>8	>8	>8	>7	>7	>7
WOMEN	1	<5	<5	<4	<3	<3	<3
	2	5–8	5–8	4–7	3–7	3–7	3–7
	3	>8	>8	>7	>7	>7	>7

<=less than; >=more than

QUALITY OF LIFE QUESTIONNAIRE

Use the number scale to answer the questions, then add the numbers to find your total.

1	2	3	4	5
Not at All	Slightly	Moderately	Quite a Bit	Extremely

During the past 4 weeks, to what extent has your joint health or concern about your health interfered with the following?

a. Your normal social activities with family, friends, neighbors, or groups ☐

b. Your general happiness ☐

c. Your ability to accomplish the tasks you have set out to do ☐

d. Your ability to perform tasks effectively and carefully ☐

Total Score ▢

Check your total score against the key below to find your level for quality of life.

16–20	8–15	4–7
Level 1	**Level 2**	**Level 3**

PHYSICAL ACTIVITY TEST

Staying physically active is one of the most important ways to maintain health, including joint health. How active are you?

Review the levels of physical activity described in the Code for Physical Activity that follows and determine which most closely describes your average level of activity during the past month. The levels range from very sedentary (1) to very active (7). Record the number that best matches your activity level on your Joint Health Profile Card. Isn't that simple?

CODE FOR PHYSICAL ACTIVITY

Choose the number (0–7) that best describes your general activity level for the previous month.

I do not participate regularly in programmed recreational sport or heavy physical activity.

☐ **0** I avoid walking or exertion—e.g., I always use an elevator and drive whenever possible instead of walking.

☐ **1** I walk for pleasure, routinely use stairs, occasionally exercise sufficiently to cause heavy breathing or perspiration.

I participate regularly in recreation or work requiring modest physical activity, such as golf, horseback riding, calisthenics, gymnastics, table tennis, bowling, weight lifting, or yard work.

☐ **2** 10 to 60 minutes per week

☐ **3** More than an hour per week

I participate regularly in heavy physical exercise, such as brisk walking, running or jogging, swimming, cycling, rowing, skipping rope, or running in place, or I engage in vigorous aerobic activity, such as tennis, basketball, or handball.

☐ **4** I run or briskly walk less than 1 mile per week or spend less than 30 minutes per week in comparable physical activity.

☐ **5** I run or briskly walk 1 to 5 miles per week or spend 30 to 60 minutes per week in comparable physical activity.

☐ **6** I run or briskly walk 5 to 10 miles per week or spend 1 to 3 hours per week in comparable physical activity.

☐ **7** I run or briskly walk more than 10 miles per week or spend more than 3 hours per week in comparable physical activity.

SOURCE: Adapted from *Exercise Concepts, Calculations and Computer Applications*, by R. M. Ross and A. S. Jackson (Dubuque, Ia.: Brown and Benchmak, 1990). Used with permission of the authors.

BODY MASS INDEX

Because being overweight is one of the major stressors of your joints, you need to evaluate your level of body fat. Your joints, your heart, and your overall health benefit from maintaining a healthy weight. Body mass index (BMI), a research tool that is used to estimate body fat, has been proven to correlate accurately to body fat and is much more accurate than the height/weight tables you may be familiar with.

The computation of BMI is based on the fact that height, weight, and body surface are related to one another. The computation uses the formula of body weight in kilograms divided by height in meters squared, but most of us skip the math and just consult a Body Mass Index Table like the one on page 50. Here's how to use it.

1. Find your height in inches in the left-hand column.
2. Run your finger horizontally across the page from this number until you find your weight in pounds.
3. Look at the bottom of the weight column to determine your BMI.
4. Record your BMI on your Joint Health Profile Card.

Judging where your BMI places you is simple.

■ A healthy BMI is between 19 and 24.9. If you fall in that range—great! You are Level 3.
■ You are overweight if your BMI is between 25 and 29.9. You are Level 2.
■ You are clinically obese if your BMI is 30 or over. You are Level 1.

INTERPRETING YOUR TEST RESULTS

The results of these tests will give you a good idea of the current status of your joint health. The tests also correlate with programs that you will find in the rest of the chapters in this section. If most of your scores put you in Level 1, you will generally want to work in the programs that are designated as red. These are the programs that are designed for people who already have some degree of joint problems or who need the most work to improve their joint health.

If most of your results put you in Level 2, you will generally want to work with those programs that are designated as yellow. As with a traffic light, yellow means caution. Although your joint health is average, you still have some way to go to achieve truly healthy joints. The yellow level programs are more vigorous than those in the red level, but not as vigorous as those in the green category.

If most of your results put you in Level 3, you will want to focus on the programs designated as green. A majority of Level 3 results on your tests means that your joints are in generally good health. The programs are designed to further enhance your joint health so that you can continue to enjoy your active life for years to come.

Mixing and matching your program. If you are like most people, you will discover that your levels in the various test areas are different. For example, you may achieve a Level 2 on the 6-minute walk but only a Level 1 on the strength and flexibility tests. That's fine. You can and should mix and match levels of activities within the 8-Week Joint Health Program to fit your exact needs.

USING YOUR PROFILE CARD TO PLAN YOUR ACTIVITIES

Once you have completed all the tests, here's how to use your Joint Health Profile Card to plan your 8-Week Joint Health Program.

Walking or other aerobic program. Look at your results for the 6-minute walk, the 50-foot walk, and the knees and hips sections of the joint health index. Are all your levels the same? If so, that's the level at which to start your walking program. Do you have a mixture of levels? If so, which level predominates? Start there with the programs in chapter 5. (You will also notice that each level has two programs, one for people age 70 and over and one for those ages 30 to 69.)

Increasing physical activity. Most people are not as active as they ought to be. If you judged your activity at Level 1 or 2, you'll want to focus on the suggestions in chapter 6 as well as on the walking programs in chapter 5.

Flexibility and strength. To determine where to start your stretching for flexibility in chapter 7, look at your results in both the joint health index and the sit-and-reach test. Consider the two results together to decide where to start. Your results may suggest that you start at different levels for upper body and lower body. Use the hand-stretch

(continued on page 54)

BODY MASS INDEX

HEIGHT (in)	WEIGHT (lb)						
58	91	95	100	105	110	114	119
59	94	99	104	109	114	119	124
60	97	102	107	112	117	122	127
61	101	106	111	117	122	127	132
62	103	109	114	120	125	130	136
63	107	113	119	124	130	135	141
64	111	117	123	129	135	141	146
65	114	120	126	132	138	144	150
66	118	124	131	137	143	149	156
67	121	127	134	140	147	153	159
68	125	132	139	145	152	158	165
69	128	135	142	149	155	162	169
70	133	140	147	154	161	168	175
71	136	143	150	157	164	171	179
72	140	148	155	162	170	177	185
73	143	151	158	166	174	181	189
74	148	156	164	171	179	187	195
75	151	159	167	175	183	191	199
76	156	164	172	181	189	197	205
BMI	**19**	**20**	**21**	**22**	**23**	**24**	**25**

SOURCE: From *Weighing the Options* (Washington, D.C.: National Academy of Sciences, 1995). Used with permission.

124	129	133	138	143	148	152	157	162
129	134	139	144	149	154	159	164	169
132	138	143	148	153	158	163	168	173
138	143	148	154	159	164	169	175	180
141	147	152	158	163	168	174	179	185
147	152	158	164	169	175	181	186	192
152	158	164	170	176	182	187	193	199
156	162	168	174	180	186	192	198	204
162	168	174	180	187	193	199	205	212
166	172	178	185	191	198	204	210	217
172	178	185	191	198	205	211	218	224
176	182	189	196	203	209	216	223	230
182	189	196	203	210	217	224	231	237
186	193	200	207	214	221	229	236	243
192	199	207	214	221	229	236	244	251
196	204	211	219	226	234	241	249	257
203	210	218	226	234	242	249	257	265
207	215	223	231	239	247	255	263	271
214	222	230	238	246	255	263	271	279
26	**27**	**28**	**29**	**30**	**31**	**32**	**33**	**34**

(continued)

BODY MASS INDEX (cont.)

HEIGHT (in)	WEIGHT (lb)							
58	167	172	176	181	186	191	195	
59	174	179	184	188	193	198	203	
60	178	183	188	194	199	204	209	
61	185	191	196	201	207	212	217	
62	190	196	201	206	212	217	223	
63	198	203	209	214	220	226	231	
64	205	211	217	223	228	234	240	
65	210	216	222	228	234	240	246	
66	218	224	230	236	243	249	255	
67	223	229	236	242	248	255	261	
68	231	238	244	251	257	264	271	
69	236	243	250	257	263	270	277	
70	244	251	258	265	272	279	286	
71	250	257	264	271	279	286	293	
72	258	266	273	281	288	295	303	
73	264	272	279	287	294	302	309	
74	273	281	288	296	304	312	319	
75	279	287	294	302	310	318	326	
76	287	296	304	312	320	328	337	
BMI	**35**	**36**	**37**	**38**	**39**	**40**	**41**	

200	205	210	214	219	224	229	233	238
208	213	218	223	228	233	238	243	248
214	219	224	229	234	239	244	250	255
222	228	233	238	244	249	254	260	265
228	234	239	245	250	255	261	266	272
237	243	248	254	260	265	271	277	282
246	252	258	264	269	275	281	287	293
252	258	264	270	276	282	288	294	300
261	268	274	280	286	292	299	305	311
268	274	280	287	293	299	306	312	319
277	284	290	297	304	310	317	323	330
284	290	297	304	311	317	324	331	338
293	300	307	314	321	328	335	342	349
300	307	314	321	329	336	343	350	357
313	317	325	332	340	347	354	362	369
317	324	332	340	347	355	362	370	377
327	335	343	351	358	366	374	382	390
334	342	350	358	366	374	382	390	398
345	353	361	370	378	386	394	402	411
42	**43**	**44**	**45**	**46**	**47**	**48**	**49**	**50**

test and the fingers portion of the joint health index to determine your dexterity program. Use the results of the leg-extension strength test and the joint health index to determine which of the strength programs in chapter 7 is the right place to begin.

Body weight. If your BMI places you in the overweight or obese category, you should focus your attention on chapters 8 and 9 in addition to beginning a walking program.

Quality of life. Think of these results as a motivating tool. Sometimes, we have to stop and take a conscious look at how joint health or lack of it is affecting our quality of life. If your joint health is having a negative impact, the whole 8-Week Joint Health Program can help. In particular, both aerobic exercise such as walking and increased general physical activity help to elevate mood, fight depression, and make you feel better about life.

READY, SET, GO!

Taking the self-evaluation tests, reading through the activities of the 8-Week Joint Health Program, and planning your program can really fire your enthusiasm. New possibilities are calling, so you tie on your walking shoes, charge out the door, and start up the hill. May I insert a word of caution here? As you plan and then start, think like a tortoise, not like a hare. In improving or enhancing joint health, the race does not usually go to the swift, so err on the side of caution by starting at a lower level in the programs. You can always increase the level quickly if it's too easy, but if you start too fast, discomfort and even injury can sabotage your efforts. Above all, remember that your goal is health and enjoyment of life, so have fun in your program.

Follow these guidelines and then, at the end of 8 weeks, take the tests again. You will be amazed at how much progress you have made toward achieving lasting joint health!

JOINT HEALTH PROFILE CARD

	Test	BASELINE		8 WEEKS		16 WEEKS	
		Results	Level	Results	Level	Results	Level
Joint health index	Knees and hips						
	Fingers						
	Back and neck						
6-minute walk							
50-foot walk							
Hand stretch							
Sit and reach							
Leg extension							
Quality of life							
Physical activity							
Body mass index							

NOTES

Each time you take the joint tests, use this page to record your thoughts about your progress.

Walking

After about age 1, when we human beings learn the skill of walking, we depend on our legs to move us about our environment, taking us wherever we need and want to go. Walking soon becomes as automatic as seeing, hearing, or breathing—and almost as important. Everyone wants to keep maximum mobility for a lifetime, and maximum mobility depends on healthy joints.

Fortunately, walking regularly or engaging in some other form of aerobic exercise offers you one of the best ways to keep your joints functioning well for many years. Even people who have osteoarthritis can improve the health and function of their joints by participating in appropriate exercise. In fact, because of the strong consensus about the multiple benefits of exercise for both the joints and general good health, recent guidelines from the Arthritis Foundation and the American College of Rheumatology emphasize gentle exercise, such as walking, as one of the key ways to improve joint health. So even if you already have some pain or problems with your knees or hips (or other joints), you can enjoy the benefits of walking or another low-impact aerobic activity, such as cycling or swimming, by taking a few extra precautions.

But wait, there's more! Beyond helping your joints stay trouble-free, walking and other forms of aerobic exercise also provide tremendous benefits for your overall health and fitness. These benefits are so numerous that I've given you a brief rundown in "Health Benefits of Aerobic Exercise" on page 58.

As the ancient Chinese proverb says, "the longest journey begins with a single step." So let's shake a leg and get started on your journey to a lifetime of joint health! I'll show you how to start a walking program

Health Benefits of Aerobic Exercise

Beyond its benefits for joints, aerobic exercise such as walking improves general health in many ways.

- It reduces the risk of heart disease. People who are regularly active throughout their lives cut their risk of heart disease in half. In other words, if you *choose* to be inactive, you double your risk of heart disease, as much as if you smoked a pack of cigarettes a day.
- It improves total cholesterol levels and elevates levels of HDL (good cholesterol).
- It lowers the risk of high blood pressure and helps to lower and control existing high blood pressure.
- It reduces the risk of diabetes and improves the body's handling of glucose in people with type 2 (non-insulin-dependent) diabetes.
- It improves bone health and reduces the risk of osteoporosis.
- It enhances weight loss, helps to maintain a healthy weight, and helps to prevent loss of lean muscle during weight loss.
- It lowers the risk of certain cancers, such as breast cancer and colon cancer.

geared to your level of fitness and joint health as well as how to adapt the walking programs to activities such as bicycling or swimming, if you prefer one of them or would like to cross-train with another activity.

LESS PAIN, MORE GAIN: THE MANY BENEFITS OF AEROBIC EXERCISE

In the past 10 years, multiple studies have consistently shown that by exercising appropriately, people decrease their joint pain and increase their strength, endurance, range of motion, and flexibility. A lot of these benefits come from increased elasticity of the connective tissue.

In addition, regular aerobic exercise seems to improve the overall nutrition of every element of the joint by promoting increased movement of synovial fluid, which stimulates and repairs cartilage. People who have joint discomfort or arthritis often notice decreased swelling in their joints after becoming involved in regular exercise programs.

Maintaining proper muscle tone and weight control through walking programs also lowers the risk of joint disease. From a functional standpoint, following a regular walking program improves your walking speed (very important as you grow older) and walking gait (which prevents falls) and lets you more easily carry out the activities of daily living.

Walking has also been shown to decrease the likelihood of disabilities throughout life as well as to improve the quality of life and general health status.

WHY WALKING?

There are many different forms of aerobic exercise, but I am a big fan of walking. In fact, my center has been the leading walking research laboratory in the United States for the past 20 years. Why am I so enthusiastic? Simply because walking is the most practical and best choice for most people.

- It is convenient and as easy as stepping outside your front door.
- It is very flexible. People of all fitness levels can walk safely and enjoyably.
- It is low-impact. Because one foot is in contact with the ground at all times, the impact of walking is very low, no more than 1 to 1¼ times your body weight.
- It is very social. People at different fitness levels and of different ages can walk together.
- Because it is convenient and low-impact, walking is the form of exercise most recommended by physicians for general health and fitness as well as for joint health. In various surveys, 90 percent of physicians put walking at the top of their recommended activities lists.

Although I will give you some guidance for other activities, it's clear from this list that as a choice for lifelong healthy joints, walking is hard to beat.

WALKING AROUND PAIN

Even if you have trouble with your joints, walking or other aerobic activity can work wonders for you. If you already have some degree of joint pain or even joint disease, such as arthritis, you should seek the advice of your own physician or physical therapist to help you plan how to start a walking program without making your condition worse. In some instances, using a cane may be helpful. It is also important not to carry heavy loads while you are walking, and *never* use hand or arm weights, because they can make arthritis and other joint problems worse. If you have joint pain, a pair of high-quality walking shoes that provide good cushioning is an absolute necessity. In fact, that's good advice for everyone.

Some people worry that a regular walking program could actually hurt their joints, making future joint problems more likely. The opposite is true. Studies of runners who log 40 to 50 miles a week have shown that their likelihood of disability is significantly less than that of people who are sedentary. One series of studies of long-distance runners and swimmers showed that even after many years of these activities, only about 2 percent had any joint problems. This rate is significantly less than that found in the general population. So don't worry—you can exercise to both your heart's and your joints' content without increasing your risk of joint problems.

Of course, there are a few exceptions to this rule. In some cases, poor technique can increase your risk of injury, so be sure to pay careful attention to the instructions with my programs. If you have any doubts, consult a trained exercise professional or physical therapist. Some sports, particularly contact sports such as football and sports that require quick turns, twists, and pivots, may increase your likelihood of future joint problems. (For more on these sports-related concerns, see chapter 16.)

BUILDING A PROGRAM

Now that you know the benefits of walking and aerobic exercise, it's time to put together your own 8-week program. Here are the basics.

GEARING UP

Even though walking is, by its nature, a simple activity, several items will increase your pleasure and safety. This is particularly true if you already have joint problems.

Good walking shoes. If you buy only one item to start your program, purchase good shoes designed specifically for fitness walking. (Yes, shoes for fitness walking and those for running are different because the mechanics of how your feet and legs operate are different in each activity.) Walking shoes must have good stability, good support, and appropriate cushioning for even the low impact of walking. Using the right shoes can help prevent strain and injury. Any good general shoe store or athletic shoe store should be able to help you select good-quality walking shoes to fit your feet. Currently, there are 10 to 15 manufacturers of excellent walking shoes in the United States.

Other gear. If stylin' down the avenue is important to you, you can purchase many different kinds of equipment even for a sport as simple as walking. I consider an all-weather exercise suit essential so that you will not be held back when it is raining, windy, or cold. Other useful gear might include a pedometer, a walking stick, or an electronic heart rate monitor (more about those later). I will leave that up to your imagination.

Leave them in the store. I do not recommend walking with hand or ankle weights, because they can lead to injury even if you do not already have joint problems. For upper-body exercises, use our stretching and strength programs. If you'd like to combine upper- and lower-body strength training with aerobics, try swimming and other water exercises.

EXERCISING SAFELY

When patients starting an exercise program ask me what the most important key to safety is, I tell them, "Don't leave your common sense behind!" By this I mean that you should always be alert to any discomfort or pain, which is nature's signal of a problem. Pain may indicate a joint problem or a larger one. Pain in your chest or both legs, for example, could indicate a problem with your heart. Always take any form of pain seriously. Pain is not a natural companion to exercise. If you have significant pain in any joint—and especially if you have pain in your chest—while walking, you should immediately consult a physician. If you've been sedentary, a little muscle soreness when you start walking may be normal, but it's also telling you not to rush. Build up intensity and duration gradually, as the programs indicate.

Do you need a checkup? Before starting your program, you may want to use the same impetus that got you thinking about an exercise regimen to have a full evaluation by your physician. A phone call may be enough to get clearance, or the doctor may want to see you. In some instances, your physician may even want you to walk on a treadmill while being monitored. This type of exercise stress test is excellent not only for determining if your heart is in good shape but also for determining your fitness level.

If you have an existing problem with either your hip or your knee, you may want to ask for a referral to a physical therapist. A therapist can help you design a specific program of exercises in conjunction with your walking program so that you can get the benefits of increased aerobic activity without aggravating any existing joint problem.

What if you have a condition such as heart disease? If you have heart disease, high blood pressure, diabetes, or another medical condition, you should consult your physician about your intended walking program. Walking programs are appropriate for most people with these conditions, and, in fact, your physician has probably recommended such a program to you. The walking programs in this chapter are generally appropriate for everyone, but be sure to follow any specific precautions that your physician gives you.

PRINCIPLES OF EFFECTIVE EXERCISE

The 8-Week Walking Program is based on the exercise principles recommended by the American College of Sports Medicine (ACSM), the source of widely accepted standards for building fitness programs, as well as on many research studies at my institute. The ACSM has shown that the most effective exercise programs are based on the principles of frequency, intensity, and time. Together, they go by the highly appropriate acronym FIT. Let's look at each of these parameters.

Frequency: how often you exercise. For most people, walking four or five times a week is optimum. Some people find that their walking programs are so enjoyable that they like to do them five or six times a week. I always recommend that you take at least 1 day a week to rest in order to allow your joints to recover. In all levels of the 8-week program, you start gradually and work up.

Intensity: how hard you exercise. Intensity is a very important parameter. Often, people exercise too hard as they start an exercise program. Walking too hard or too fast too soon can lead to soreness, injury, and quitting. To judge how hard you're walking, take the talk test. When you are walking, you should be able to carry on a conversation at a normal level. You should not be able to shout or sing opera, but you should be able to talk in normal tones. If you are too short of breath to talk, you are exercising too hard. For most people, the talk test will help them get in the right range.

You can also accurately judge how hard you are exercising by using the Revised Borg Scale of Rate of Perceived Exertion (RPE). Using a scale of 1 to 10, you can accurately estimate the intensity of your workout from nothing at all to very, very strong. My walking programs use intensity levels from moderate (3) and somewhat strong (4) to strong (5) and very strong (7).

REVISED BORG SCALE OF RATE OF PERCEIVED EXERTION (RPE)

0	Nothing at all
0.5	Very, very weak
1	Very weak
2	Weak
3	Moderate
4	Somewhat strong
5	Strong
6	
7	Very strong
8	
9	
10	Very, very strong
11	

Another good way to determine intensity is to use a target heart rate. I recommend a target of 50 to 70 percent of your predicted maximum heart rate. To determine your predicted maximum, subtract your age in years from 220 beats per minute. Then, to determine the lower end of your target heart rate range, divide your predicted maximum rate in half. To determine the upper end of the range, divide your predicted maximum rate by 10 and then multiply by 7. If you wish to use target heart-rate, I recommend that you use a portable electronic heart-rate monitor. Accurate monitors are now relatively inexpensive and provide a good way to stay in your target zone and stay motivated.

Time: how long you exercise. I recommend that you build up to approximately 30 minutes of aerobic exercise each day that you exercise. This expert recommendation comes from a review of hundreds of research studies performed under the direction of the Centers for Disease Control and Prevention. The good news is that rather than getting your 30 minutes all at once, you can accumulate 30 minutes of moderate-intensity walking over the course of the day.

COMPONENTS OF AN AEROBIC
EXERCISE PROGRAM

All good aerobic exercise programs consist of three components—warmup, exercise, and cooldown. Each session of the 8-Week Walking Program emphasizes these three activities.

Warmup. This is a period of 5 to 7 minutes in which you do stretching and light exercise, such as walking, to warm up the musculoskeletal and cardiovascular systems for more intense exercise. Use stretches from your level of the 8-Week Stretching Program presented in chapter 7.

Aerobic component. During this component, which typically lasts 15 to 30 minutes, you exercise at a somewhat higher rate as measured by your rate of perceived exertion or your target heart rate. The types of aerobic exercise programs that have been shown to be safe and effective for improving joint health include walking, swimming, stationary cycling, and water exercise.

Cooldown. For safety and comfort, doing a cooldown is as important as doing a warmup. After completing the aerobic component, spend 5 to 7 minutes gradually cooling down and stretching. In fact, because your muscles are thoroughly warmed up from exercising, the cooldown is a good time to perform the stretching exercises presented in chapter 7. If you have time to do just one or two, select those for the lower body.

THE 8-WEEK WALKING PROGRAM

Presented on the following pages are the three levels of the 8-Week Walking Program—red, yellow, and green. The least intense are the Level 1 red programs, the Level 2 yellow programs are moderate, and the most intense are the Level 3 green programs. Which level of walking program is right for you to begin? Use your Joint Health Profile Card as instructed in chapter 4 to decide.

You will notice that there are two programs for the first two levels—

one for people ages 30 to 69 and the other for those age 70 and over. For Level 3, the program is the same for all ages, and at all three levels, men and women use the same program because the use of appropriate intensity fits the program to individual needs.

I have also included pace, but unless you use a pedometer, this is not a category that you need to worry about. If you walk for the indicated length of time at the intensity recommended, you will be walking at about the pace indicated.

When you complete the first 8-week program, test your progress using the 6-minute walk test and either repeat the program or move to the next level if you're ready. When you complete Level 3, you can maintain your walking program at this level. If you find that you want to progress even further, you may want to consult my book *Fit over Forty*, which gives more advanced walking programs and a diet plan for weight loss. For variety, you may also wish to mix in cross-training with other aerobic activities.

RED WALKING PROGRAM (LEVEL 1—AGE 70+)

	WEEK							
	1	2	3	4	5	6	7	8
Frequency (days)	3	4	4	4	4	5	5	5
Warmup (min)	3	3	5	5	5–7	5–7	5–7	5–7
Pace (mph)	1.7	2.0	2.0	2.0	2.0	2.5	2.5	2.0
Time walked (min)	10	10	15	18	18	18	18	20
RPE* or heart rate (% of max)	3 50–60	3 50–60	3–4 50–60	4 60	4 60	4–5 60–70	4–5 60–70	5 60–70
Cooldown (min)	3	3	5	5	5–7	5–7	5–7	5–7

*Rate of perceived exertion

RED WALKING PROGRAM (LEVEL 1—AGES 30–69)

	WEEK							
	1	2	3	4	5	6	7	8
Frequency (days)	3	4	4	4	4	5	5	5
Warmup (min)	3	3	5	5	5–7	5–7	5–7	5–7
Pace (mph)	2.2	2.5	2.5	2.5	2.7	3.0	3.0	3.0
Time walked (min)	10	10	15	18	18	18	18	20
RPE* or heart rate (% of max)	3–4 50–60	3–4 50–60	4 60	4 60–70	4–5 60–70	5 60–70	5–6 60–70	5–6 60–70
Cooldown (min)	3	3	5	5	5–7	5–7	5–7	5–7

*Rate of perceived exertion

YELLOW WALKING PROGRAM (LEVEL 2—AGE 70+)

	WEEK							
	1	2	3	4	5	6	7	8
Frequency (days)	3	4	4	4	4	5	5	5
Warmup (min)	3	3	5	5	5–7	5–7	5–7	5–7
Pace (mph)	2.5	2.5	2.5	2.7	2.7	3.0	3.0	3.0
Time walked (min)	15	15	18	18	20	20	20	25
RPE* or heart rate (% of max)	4 50–60	4 50–60	4 60	4–5 60	5 60–70	5 60–70	5–6 60–70	5–6 60–70
Cooldown (min)	3	3	5	5	5–7	5–7	5–7	5–7

*Rate of perceived exertion

YELLOW WALKING PROGRAM (LEVEL 2—AGES 30–69)

	WEEK							
	1	2	3	4	5	6	7	8
Frequency (days)	3	4	4	4	4	5	5	5
Warmup (min)	3	3	5	5	5–7	5–7	5–7	5–7
Pace (mph)	3.0	3.0	3.3	3.5	3.3	3.5	3.5	3.3
Time walked (min)	15	15	18	18	20	20	20	25
RPE* or heart rate (% of max)	5 50–60	5 60	5–6 60–70	5–6 60–70	6 60–70	6 60–70	6–7 60–70	6–7 60–70
Cooldown (min)	3	3	5	5	5–7	5–7	5–7	5–7

*Rate of perceived exertion

GREEN WALKING PROGRAM (LEVEL 3—ALL AGES)

	WEEK							
	1	2	3	4	5	6	7	8
Frequency (days)	3	4	4	4	4	5	5	5
Warmup (min)	3	3	5	5	5–7	5–7	5–7	5–7
Pace (mph)	3.0	3.3	3.5	3.5	3.5	3.7	3.5	3.7
Time walked (min)	15	15	18	20	24	24	28	30
RPE* or heart rate (% of max)	5 60	5–6 60	6 60–70	6 60–70	6–7 60–70	6–7 60–70	7 60–70	7 70
Cooldown (min)	3	3	5	5	5–7	5–7	5–7	5–7

*Rate of perceived exertion

OTHER AEROBIC EXERCISES THAT PROMOTE JOINT HEALTH

Although I am very enthusiastic about regular walking as a way of building joint health, there are other forms of aerobic activity that I can recommend. You can use the FIT (frequency, intensity, time) parameters given in the 8-week walking programs for any of these other activities. For occasional variety, you can even substitute a swimming or cycling session in your walking program. Again, just use the same FIT levels.

Cycling. Cycling, whether outdoor or stationary, is an excellent form of exercise for overall joint health, particularly for people who have joint problems in their hips and knees. The great thing about cycling is that it is very low-impact. Because the cycle supports your body weight, you can exercise without any additional pounding on your bones and joints. A number of studies have shown that cycling can improve joint health.

If you haven't been on a bicycle lately, you may wish to begin with stationary cycling or at least cycling only on level surfaces until you refine your skills and build up your stamina. Remember to always wear a safety helmet when cycling outdoors.

Swimming. Swimming is also excellent for promoting joint health. The water supports your weight, so you get a terrific cardiovascular and muscular workout with minimum adverse impact on the bones and joints.

Water exercise. A variety of water exercise programs have been developed to take advantage of the body support that water offers. Most health clubs and YMCAs have good programs of water exercise. These types of exercises are particularly beneficial for people who already have arthritis or other joint problems. If you have any questions, you can contact a local health club to find out what types of water exercise programs are offered there.

Other exercises. Other forms of aerobic exercise, such as aerobic dance, step aerobics, or running, may also be appropriate for certain people who are seeking to improve their joint health. If you already have joint problems, however, you should be very careful about participating in these activities, because they are high-impact. The extra pounding and stress can aggravate any joint problems that you already have. Although some physicians recommend machine rowing as a low-impact exercise, I caution against it. Poorly designed equipment (most inexpensive rowing machines) and poor technique (common without trained instruction) pose a great danger of strain and injury. I would recommend against choosing rowing unless you are under the direct supervision of a physical therapist.

Remember that "the longest journey begins with a single step." Are you ready? It's time to open that front door and take your first step toward a lifetime of joint-friendly fitness walking!

Getting More Activity Every Day

Of course, there are no magic cures or preventives in medicine or any other aspect of life—but physical activity comes close. Human beings were designed to move; it is only as our world has become increasingly mechanized and computerized that we have forgotten this. If you asked me to make just one recommendation to improve your joint health and your general health, I'd say to increase your physical activity until you reach and maintain a 6 or 7 on the Code for Physical Activity that you used for self-evaluation in chapter 4. Physical activity is unquestionably one of the best health promoters that each of us can incorporate into our daily lives.

A few years ago, I served on a panel of 14 experts called together to advise the Centers for Disease Control and Prevention (CDC), whose mandate is to look after the health and well-being of all citizens in the United States, about physical activity. After months of reviewing and correlating hundreds of previous studies and deliberating intensely, our panel made some simple but major recommendations. Basically, we urged all adults in the United States to try to accumulate at least 30 minutes of moderate physical activity on most, if not all, days.

The panel's recommendations were published in the *Journal of the American Medical Association* in an article titled "Physical Activity and Public Health: Recommendations from the Centers for Disease Control and Prevention and the American College of Sports Medicine." They became the basis for the *Surgeon General's Report on Physical Activity and Health*—and they can also become the basis for your improved health.

The operative words in our basic recommendation are *accumulate* and *moderate*. By "accumulate," we mean that all of the physical activity does not have to occur at one time. You could take a 10-minute walk in the morning, garden for 15 minutes in the afternoon, and intermittently take the stairs throughout the day, and you would satisfy the requirements for accumulating 30 minutes of physical activity on any given day. "Moderate" activity is more vigorous than light activity but less than strenuous. Moderately intense fitness walking fits into this category, and so does energetic outdoor gardening.

Among the many health benefits that these guidelines foster is improved and sustained joint health. As you will see, I advocate all kinds of physical activity to benefit not just joint health but also total well-being. While I'm going to show you how to look for opportunities for increased activity that you may have overlooked or underestimated, I want to emphasize the benefits and joys of gardening.

Why do I single out gardening? The answer is simple. Over the years, I have noticed that my patients who are gardeners tend to have much better health than other patients do. My observation is supported by several studies that show that people who garden regularly lower their risk of chronic disease. The physical activity involved clearly produces some physical health benefits, but just as important, gardening fosters a particularly wonderful mind/body relationship. Over and above the physical benefits, gardeners derive a host of spiritual benefits from being connected to the earth, even when the earth is contained in pots on a windowsill or patio.

GOOD NEWS FOR YOUR JOINTS

Here's the bottom line about physical activity: People who are physically active throughout their lives usually have healthier joints than their sedentary peers. The benefits of moderate, accumulated physical activity are very similar to those provided by a regular program of walking or other aerobic activity, as discussed in chapter 5. Depending on the activity, however, the benefits may extend to a much wider range of joints than they may with walking. People who are involved in regular gardening, lawn care, or housework, for example, can derive benefits for arthritic hands, elbows, and shoulders.

Like walking and other aerobic exercise, accumulated, moderate physical activity benefits your joints in the following ways.

- It helps all of the elements of the joint structure, such as cartilage and bone, maintain the proper nourishment for good health.
- It strengthens muscles and maintains good muscle tone.
- It reduces symptoms of joint problems, such as pain or stiffness.
- It increases strength and endurance.
- It improves range of motion and flexibility.
- It improves the flexibility and elasticity of all of the connective tissues that are integral to a healthy joint.

Even more important than aerobic activity, regular physical activity increases your capacity to carry out the functions and activities of daily living. A study performed in my laboratory a few years ago looked at the physical capacity of more than 340 people between the ages of 40 and 80. It showed that those who were physically active had significantly improved balance, strength, and aerobic capacity, all of which make it possible to live a vigorous, full life. When it comes to your joints, the phrase "use it or lose it" clearly applies. By using joints in healthy ways through increased physical activity, we are using them for their intended function, which, in a wonderful natural cycle, strengthens their ability to keep fulfilling that function. The regularly active subjects in my study also showed improved mood, indicated by less depression and anxiety and improved quality of life. By their very nature, many forms of physical activity are also social activities that foster personal interaction. All of these contribute to good health.

Because it nurtures joint health and the other factors that strengthen balance, mobility, and functioning, physical activity is *the* key that unlocks the door to joyful, independent, active living for all of our days.

A BOOST FOR YOUR OVERALL HEALTH

Of course, if you have healthy joints but the rest of your body is breaking down, life won't be so fine. Here again, physical activity is the answer—the nearest thing modern medicine has to a magic cure or preventive. There is almost nothing bad about physical activity, particularly if you use common sense and a few safety precautions while pursuing your favorite activities.

To put in perspective how much you stand to gain, let me tell you about a major study that the CDC published a few years ago. This particular study compared the risk of developing heart disease in people who had "active" lifestyles with the risk of those who had "inactive" lifestyles. Applying statistical methods to the data from 43 previous, scientifically rigorous studies, the scientists at the CDC concluded that people who were physically active throughout their lives had half the risk of heart disease of inactive people. The investigators concluded that the choice to lead an inactive life predisposes people to the same increased risk as smoking a pack of cigarettes a day. Unfortunately, by CDC criteria, more than 60 percent of the population in the United States is inactive.

In addition to lowering your risk of heart disease, regular moderate physical activity offers the same specific benefits for health that I presented in "Health Benefits of Aerobic Exercise" on page 58. If you need a reminder, go back and check these out.

HOW MUCH IS ENOUGH?

Sometimes, people are confused about what is meant by light and moderate activity. To help reduce the confusion, the CDC's expert panel put together lists of activities that would be regarded as light, moderate, and vigorous (see "Intensity Levels of Common Activities" on page 74).

Most of the activities that fall into the light and moderate categories are fairly simple to perform. Some of them involve the kinds of aerobic activities that I discussed in chapter 5, but many also involve everyday activities, such as gardening and various household tasks. To help stimulate your thinking about forms of activity that you can accumulate in your own life, let's look first at gardening, with its wide range of potential joint-healthy activities.

YEAR-ROUND BENEFITS FROM GARDENING

Those of us who are already gardeners don't need to be convinced that this is a wonderful activity. As a method of improving joint health, how-

INTENSITY LEVELS OF COMMON ACTIVITIES

LIGHT	MODERATE	VIGOROUS/HARD
Walking slowly (1–2 mph)	Walking briskly (3–4 mph)	Walking briskly with a load
Stationary cycling (less than 50 rpm)	Cycling for pleasure or transportation (<10 mph)	Cycling fast (>10 mph)
Swimming slowly	Swimming with moderate effort	Swimming fast
Light stretching	General calisthenics	——
Golf, using power cart	Golf, pulling cart/carrying clubs	——
——	Table tennis	Singles racquetball
Bowling	——	——
Fishing, sitting	Fishing, standing/casting	Fishing in stream
Boating, in power boat	Canoeing leisurely	Canoeing rapidly
Vacuuming carpet	General housecleaning	Moving furniture
Mowing lawn, using riding mower	Mowing lawn, using power push mower	Mowing lawn, using hand push mower
Carpentry	Painting house	——

ever, gardening is vastly underrated. Gardening is a wonderful combination of physical activity that nourishes the body and emotional activity that nourishes the mind. Gardeners are, by their very nature, optimists. We plant seeds in the spring, lovingly tend our plants throughout the growing season, and then bring in a bounty of fruits, vegetables, or flowers.

Gardening can be a four-season, year-round endeavor. Each turn of the calendar brings new and varied activities. Myriad tasks require different types of light, moderate, and, if you choose, vigorous activity that exercises muscles and joints. Gardening presents multiple opportunities daily to accumulate a little activity here and there. One famous landscape architect, for instance, takes his morning cup of coffee into the garden, where he nips off faded blossoms for as long as the cup and a refill last. Here are some ways that you can enjoy the benefits gardening offers—sometimes, even if you don't have a garden.

FOUR SEASONS OF PLEASURABLE ACTIVITY

To demonstrate just how much gardening offers, I put Vivaldi's *Four Seasons* on the CD player for a little inspiration and brainstormed the following list. Of course, this is a very personal list, and every activity won't be right for your geographical area or particular garden, but you can build on these ideas.

Spring

- Prepare a new bed for vegetables or flowers, breaking ground by hand with a digging fork and spade or power tilling the first time and turning in compost by hand.
- Till established beds by hand.
- Divide perennials.
- Prune ornamental and border grasses (such as liriope) before spring budding.
- Prune spring-blooming shrubs after flowering is over.
- Plant seeds and bedding plants.
- Thin seedlings.
- Dethatch the lawn by hand.
- Lime and fertilize the lawn.
- Dig dandelions the old-fashioned way, with a long-handled weed puller; 10-minute sessions are good exercise, and no herbicides are needed.
- Hike in a nearby state park or national forest to enjoy spring wildflowers.
- Take in a flower show.

Summer

- Weed, weed, weed—take out your frustrations in a daily 10- to 15-minute session.
- For longer weeding sessions, use a long-handled scuffle hoe to exercise your arms and save your knees and back.

- Stake growing vegetables and flowers.
- Mow the lawn with a push power mower.
- Take grass clippings to the compost pile in several trips.
- Pick flowers and harvest vegetables; share with friends.
- Trim hedges and shrubs.
- Deadhead faded blossoms for a few minutes daily.
- Visit a botanical garden; stop and smell the roses.
- Plant fall vegetables—lettuce, broccoli, cauliflower, brussels sprouts, and greens.
- Make root cuttings of geraniums, impatiens, coleus, and other flowers that you'd like to enjoy over winter as houseplants.

Autumn

- Plant spring bulbs.
- Rake leaves, then rake some more; try out one of the new ergonomically designed hand rakes.
- Compost those leaves.
- Clean out dead and dying plants in flowerbeds and vegetable gardens.
- Mulch flowerbeds for winter.
- Take a hike in the woods to enjoy the fall foliage.
- Divide perennials.
- Turn under winter weeds in the vegetable garden; sow winter cover or mulch.
- Plant pansies, snapdragons, and other overwintering annuals (in milder climates).

Winter

- Plan next season's garden while riding your stationary bike.
- Take soil samples.
- Clean and repair garden paths, walks, and furniture.
- Clean and repair garden tools.
- Install new garden features, such as paths, walls, or patios.
- Build a coldframe to get a head start on the season.
- Order a kit and build a new garden bench in the garage.
- Build a trellis or arbor.
- Make garden snow sculptures with the kids.

- Hike in the winter woods; go snowshoeing or cross-country skiing.
- Prune trees the last few weeks before spring.

Clearly, a gardener's invitation to physical activity is always open.

GARDENING WITHOUT A GARDEN

But what if you don't have even a patch of earth to garden? No problem. Determined gardeners can till the soil and bring forth beauty any-where—on small city lots, on windowsills and in window boxes, in containers on decks, balconies, and patios.

I know of city dwellers whose beautiful plants cascade from every window and arrange themselves gracefully below artfully placed grow lights. Think of all that healthful oxygen, not to mention the physical activity of watering and grooming plants, rotating pots, and trekking to the plant store to bring home more.

I heard of another city dweller who grew delicious tomatoes, egg-plant, squash, and cucumbers—plus lots and lots of flowers—in containers on the rooftop deck outside her New York brownstone apartment. She also got extra physical activity as she climbed in and out through the window that gave the only access to her deck.

For a woman I knew when she was in her eighties, gardening was a source of joy and gave her opportunities to stay active and share with others. She had multiple health problems and lived in a nursing home, where she shared a single room, but she was able to garden on the tiny patio that adjoined the room and to share plants with other residents and visitors. With determination, she also took her walk around the grounds each day and was a lively thorn prodding the administrators as an unofficial ombudsman for the other patients.

My point is that neither space nor age nor any other "limitation" should stay you from pursuing gardening or whatever physical activity gives you pleasure. That activity will also help you maintain healthy, functioning joints.

TIPS FOR GARDENING SAFELY

As with any good thing, you can carry physical activity to an extreme, particularly if you've been sedentary. Remember, if you're just starting gardening or any other activity, that "moderate" applies to the length of your sessions as well as to their intensity. Don't indulge in any daylong marathons of weeding or spading, or your back and probably every joint in your body will complain. You probably won't do any lasting damage, but you might sabotage your good intentions to be more active.

In addition, there are some specific precautions that you can take to guard against harming rather than helping your joints while gardening.

- Use knee pads or kneelers, don't spend long sessions on your knees, and stretch every 10 minutes or so.
- Use good posture when performing activities such as raking, spading, and hoeing.
- Don't spade the whole flowerbed in one session if you're spading by hand; start early and do it in shorter sessions.
- Use long-handled, lightweight spades or digging tools, and don't overload them.
- Rest frequently and drink plenty of water, particularly in hot weather.
- Lift using your legs, not your back.
- Carry several small loads of trash or garden equipment instead of one large one.
- Use good tools and maintain them.
- Always wear work gloves and protective clothing.

HOW TO MAKE YOUR LIFE MORE ACTIVE

One way to put more activity, including gardening, into your life is to look objectively at how much day-to-day activity your life currently includes. Go back to your results on the physical activity test on page 47. How did you score? If you are like most American adults, you probably found that your average physical activity level puts you in the category of 0, 1, or 2. That is far too little activity. It means that your joints are not getting the nourishment and use that are required to keep them healthy and vigorous for life. It also means that you are accepting an enormous health risk for cardiovascular disease and other chronic diseases. Even categories 3, 4, and 5 are not enough. I want everyone to try to achieve category 6 or 7.

Here is the goal: Try to fit at least 30 minutes of moderate-intensity physical activity into your life on most, if not all, days. That is the level at which your joints will remain strong and lubricated and at which you will also derive other significant health benefits. It is also the point at which you will start to make a noticeable difference in your energy level and your ability to control your weight and at which you will simply feel more joy in life. The key thing here is that you don't have to turn your life upside down. To achieve this rather modest level of physical activity, all you need to do is to incorporate some common activities that you enjoy into each day's routine. Use the following five checklists to help you think about the possibilities. Then you need to use the six tips on page 81 to help you make these activities a priority.

OUTDOOR CHORES

- Chopping wood
- Cleaning gutters
- Gardening (of course!)
- Mowing
- Painting the house
- Picking up yard litter
- Raking
- Shoveling snow
- Stacking wood
- Sweeping
- Washing and waxing the car
- Washing windows

INDOOR CHORES

- Carpentry
- Cleaning
- Grocery shopping
- Painting walls
- Plastering walls
- Scraping paint from walls and trim
- Scrubbing
- Sweeping, mopping, and waxing floors
- Standing (working as a cashier, retail sales associate, or artist, for example)
- Stocking shelves
- Vacuuming and dusting
- Woodworking

LEISURE ACTIVITIES

- Archery
- Badminton
- Ballroom dancing
- Bicycling leisurely (5 mph)
- Billiards or pool
- Canoeing slowly
- Croquet
- Disco dancing
- Fishing
- Hiking (no load)

- Horse grooming
- Horseback riding
- Horseshoes
- Performing with a drill team or marching band
- Recreational table tennis
- Rowing slowly
- Sailing
- Scuba diving
- Shuffleboard
- Skating
- Skiing slowly
- Sledding
- Snowshoeing
- Square or folk dancing
- Swimming slowly
- Walking (3 mph)
- Water skiing
- Yoga

RECREATIONAL SPORTS

- Baseball (not pitching)
- Basketball (if you have no knee problems)
- Bicycle racing
- Canoe racing
- Cricket
- Fencing
- Field hockey
- Golf
- Handball
- Judo, karate, and other martial arts
- Mountain hiking and climbing
- Racquetball
- Skiing
- Soccer
- Table tennis
- Tennis
- Volleyball

ACTIVITIES FOR CARDIOVASCULAR FITNESS

- Aerobic dance (low-impact)
- Cross-country skiing (machine or actual)
- Cycling (stationary, 50 to 60 rpm; outdoor, 10 mph)
- In-line skating
- Jogging or running
- Swimming
- Walking (3 mph or more)

CHOOSING THE LEVEL THAT'S RIGHT FOR YOU

Use the overall results of the tests you took in chapter 4 to help you determine how much physical activity you want to begin with. If most of your activities or your joint symptoms put you in the red category, start with just 5 to 10 minutes of physical activity on most days. If your scores put you mostly in the yellow category, you might try 10 to 20 minutes to start. If most of your scores put you in the green category, you can jump into 20 to 30 minutes of accumulated, moderate-intensity physical activity on most, if not all, days. Remember, as I advised in the area of walking, don't leave your common sense behind. If you are experiencing any problems with your joints, be sure to have your physician or physical therapist work with you to establish the safest routine to increase your physical activity.

TIPS FOR BOOSTING YOUR ACTIVITY LEVEL

Although the preceding lists suggest many choices of activity, I know from many patients whom I have counseled in this area that it is sometimes hard to figure out exactly how to incorporate them into daily life. Over the years, I have learned many of the strategies that my patients have adopted to remind themselves of the importance of making increased activity a reality. Let me offer some of the tips that seem to be particularly helpful to them.

Accumulate, accumulate. Remember that *accumulate* is the key word. You don't have to carve out an entire half-hour at any given time. Instead, look for those small nooks and crannies in your life that present themselves as opportunities to be more active.

Specify a time and place. Most of us find that routines are helpful. If you incorporate a time for activity into your routine, you are more likely to do it. If you leave it as a low priority, you are unlikely to do it.

Have fun. My patients who set out to do activities that they described as enjoyable were much more likely to stay with them than those who regarded increasing physical activity as a grim chore.

Include family and friends. Many forms of physical activity are social activities as well, so you can include family and friends in your desire to be more active. It's another way to have fun and enjoy a little "quality time." Leave the cell phone at home!

Seize the day. Each day, look for opportunities to add activity in the normal course of your life: Take the stairs rather than the elevator. Park farther from the door of the store and walk across the parking lot. Pretty soon, you'll find that you are always on the lookout for ways to increase physical activity. You'll also save time, since in most modern buildings, taking the stairs is faster than taking the elevator!

Reward yourself. If you have succeeded in increasing your activity level, acknowledge your accomplishment. You have done one of the very best things that you can do to improve your joint health and lower your risk of chronic disease. Take the time to reward yourself by buying a CD or a book that you want, or recognize your achievement in some other way.

I have often thought of physical activity as a gift that each of us can give ourselves to maintain a healthy body for a lifetime. So get up, get out, and get going—and give yourself the gift of physical and emotional well-being!

Stretching and Strengthening

To be healthy and pain-free, your joints must have an adequate range of motion plus flexibility and strength in the muscles that surround and support them. That's why, in addition to walking and other physical activity, the 8-Week Joint Health Program includes the following:

- A stretching program that will enhance range of motion and flexibility
- A resistance, or weight-training, program that will build muscle strength
- A dexterity program that will improve flexibility and strength in the fingers and hands, which are the most common sites of osteoarthritis

Stretching and flexibility exercises to improve range of motion and strength training to help stabilize the joints and improve impact absorption are so important to joint health that they are the cornerstones of physical therapy for athletes and others who have joint injuries. This chapter offers specific 8-week programs of exercises at three levels that will enable you to use the stretching, strength training, and dexterity routines to maximize joint health and/or to improve symptoms and the function of any joint that already has problems.

BENEFITS OF IMPROVED RANGE OF MOTION AND FLEXIBILITY

Failing to maintain adequate flexibility in your muscles and joints now ultimately sets you up for later joint problems that can make it difficult to perform even simple tasks, such as getting in and out of a chair, the shower, the bed, or the car. But maintaining or increasing your flexibility yields a host of immediate and future benefits.

Enhanced joint nourishment. The normal motions of a joint promote the flow of synovial fluid around cartilage and other structures in the joint, which is essential for its proper nourishment. Flexibility is essential for normal motion.

Better joint alignment. Flexible muscles are important for proper support and alignment of joints. If muscles become stiff and weak, allowing misalignment, any predisposition to joint problems will become worse. By promoting proper alignment, adequate flexibility also strengthens the joint's ability to absorb the shock of any impact, such as running or jumping.

Injury prevention. If you lack flexibility, you are likely to have difficulty catching yourself and recovering from a fall. Stiff, inflexible joints are more susceptible to traumatic injury. In addition, there is a direct relationship between flexibility and balance that becomes more prominent as people grow older. Longitudinal studies, such as a study in Baltimore funded by the National Institutes of Health that has followed individuals over a number of decades, have established this very important relationship. Simply stated, a regular program of flexibility exercise is an excellent insurance policy against debilitating falls, particularly in older people. In addition, regular stretching exercises can prevent the type of overextension that leads to muscle pulls or tears and specific kinds of joint damage such as sprains and cartilage tears. Significantly, it is never too late to start a stretching program. In fact, recent research has shown that regular stretching can improve flexibility in people of all ages, from fortysomethings to those in their eighties and nineties.

Improved performance. Enhancing flexibility is a great way to improve your performance, whether in activities around the house or in recreational athletics. If you are an avid golfer or tennis player, for example, becoming more flexible could improve your performance in these sports. Or, if you simply want to be able to pick up your children or grandchildren, increased flexibility will make it easier and less likely to cause injury.

Increased strength. A regular stretching program is a wonderful and very underrated technique for building strength. When you relax one set of muscles during a stretch, you must contract the other, opposite muscles, which are called antagonist muscles, to hold the stretch position. This contraction builds strength in those muscles through the type of exercise called isometric.

Slowing of the aging process. Multiple studies have shown that flexibility declines with age. Some of this decline is caused by changes in the muscle, connective tissue, and other components of the joints. A much larger component of the decrease is a result of inactivity and the cultural expectation that we will become less active as we become older. If you are involved in a regular stretching program, you can slow the natural tendency of muscles and joints to become less flexible with age.

HOW FLEXIBILITY AND STRETCHING HELP JOINT PROBLEMS

Joint problems contribute to major decreases in flexibility. The resulting stiffness can significantly affect the ease of even such simple activities as rising from a chair or toilet seat or climbing a flight of stairs. Therefore, flexibility exercises are very important for people who have existing joint problems.

Let me add a word of caution, however. If you have been diagnosed as having osteoarthritis or other significant joint disease, injury, or condition, you will want to work with your physical therapist and/or physician to develop a specific set of flexibility exercises that will work best for you. The stretching exercises in this chapter are designed to be part of a good general, safe program. Nevertheless, they will need to be modified to accommodate any specific joint problems or issues that you have.

THE 8-WEEK STRETCHING PROGRAM

This program is a good general stretching regimen that starts you off slowly and progresses safely and effectively. You may use it every day whether or not you also walk or do strength training. Because it's much easier and safer to stretch muscles and tendons that are already warmed up, I recommend that you do the stretching program after you complete your walking (or other aerobic exercise) session. If you like, you may also do the complete program following your strength training.

Note: It's extremely important that you include light stretching as part of your warmup and cooldown for each walking and strength-training workout. The routine that I follow, and that I recommend for you, is to warm up with a little light exercise—3 to 4 minutes of walking or stationary cycling—then do some light stretching before beginning the major walking or strength-training session. At the end of the session, cool down with more light walking or cycling and, if you don't do your complete stretching routine then, some more light stretching. Never skip your cooldown, because it helps prevent sore muscles, and just stopping "cold" after an exercise session can sometimes trigger problems with heart rhythm.

EQUIPMENT

- Comfortable, loose clothing suitable for exercise
- Sports shoes with nonslip soles
- A straight-backed chair, such as a dining chair that doesn't roll
- A comfortable, firm surface to lie on; thick carpet is fine, but I prefer an inexpensive 1½-inch-thick exercise mat, which you can find at sporting goods stores

GENERAL GUIDELINES

1. Always warm up before and cool down after your workout.
2. Stretch slowly and breathe deeply. Don't hold your breath. Unless instructed otherwise for a specific exercise, you should stretch until you feel a gentle tugging or pulling sensation. Never stretch to the point of pain. Hold each stretch for the specified amount of time, then ease out of the stretch and back to your starting position.
3. *Never* bounce during stretches. That's called ballistic stretching, and it's a joint no-no. It can injure your joints and muscles and is not as effective as the slow, easy technique just described.
4. If you've had an injury, ask your physician to refer you to a physical therapist or exercise physiologist who can give you a program that

helps you recover safely and strengthens your joints rather than potentially hurting them further.

THE STRETCHING EXERCISES

Use these stretches for your flexibility program. Look at the chart for your level to determine the number of repetitions and the amount of time you should hold each stretch. When performed regularly and done slowly, stretching is very safe, which is why we recommend that you perform your full stretching program at least once a day, especially on days that you walk (see chapter 5).

The purpose of the program is to build flexibility as safely as possible while allowing you to make real progress. When you look at the charts, you will notice that within the program for each level, the individual exercises are also designated as L1, L2, or L3. This is to indicate that although your test scores place you in the Level 1 program, for example, you will soon advance to include some L2 and L3 exercises. These individual exercises have been incorporated into carefully graduated programs so that you can begin at the appropriate level for you and achieve your goals safely and quickly. You will also notice that as you progress through the weeks of the program, you will continue to do some exercises, while you will replace others with higher-level stretches.

L1 Stretches

Head Turns: Sit or stand with your head erect and facing forward. Turn your head slowly to look over one shoulder, hold, then slowly turn to look over the other shoulder. Keep your head level during the stretch; don't dip or roll it. Repeat as indicated.

Chin to Chest: Sit or stand with your head erect and facing forward. Lower your chin slowly to your chest. Hold, then return to the starting position, being careful not to tilt your head back when you raise it. Repeat as indicated.

Front Arm Raises: Stand straight with your arms at your sides. Slowly raise them simultaneously in front of you until they are parallel to the floor, hold, then slowly lower them back to the starting position. Repeat as indicated.

Side Arm Raises: Stand straight with your arms at your sides. Slowly raise them simultaneously out to the sides until they are parallel

(continued on page 92)

STRETCHING PROGRAM—LEVEL 1

	WEEK		
	1	2	3
Head Turns (L1)	5R; 2S	10R; 2S	10R; 5S
Chin to Chest (L1)	5R; 3S	5R; 5S	5R; 5S
Front Arm Raises (L1)	5R; 1S	10R; 1S	10R; 1S
Side Arm Raises (L1)	5R; 1S	10R; 1S	10R; 1S
Shoulder Stretches (L1)	5R; 3S	5R; 3S	5R; 3S
Side Leans (L1)	3R; 5S	5R; 5S	5R; 8S
Knee Touches (L1)	3R; 8S	5R; 8S	5R; 10S
Seated Toe Touches (L1)	3R; 5S	3R; 5S	3R; 5S
Shoulder Rolls (L2)			
Allternate Arm across Chest (L2)			
Front Arm Circles (L2)			
Side Arm Circles (L2)			
Knees to Chest (L2)			
Head Tilts (L3)			
Advanced Seated Toe Touches (L3)			
Quadriceps Stretches (L3)			
Wall Leans (L3)			
Triceps Stretches (L3)			
Butterflies (L3)			

R=repetitions; S=time to hold stretch (sec)

4	5	6	7	8
10R; 5S	10R; 5S	10R; 5S	10R; 5S	10R; 5S
5R; 5S	5R; 5S	5R; 5S	5R; 5S	5R; 5S
5R; 8S	5R; 8S	5R; 8S	5R; 8S	5R; 8S
5R; 10S	5R; 10S			
3R; 5S	3R; 5S			
5R	10R	10R	15R	15R
5R; 3S	5R; 3S	5R; 5S	5R; 5S	5R; 5S
10R	10R	15R	15R	15R
10R	10R	15R	15R	15R
		3R; 5S	5R; 5S	5R; 5S
		3R; 5S	3R; 5S	5R; 5S
		5R; 10S	5R; 10S	5R; 10S
		3R; 5S	3R; 5S	3R; 5S
		2R; 5S	3R; 5S	3R; 5S
		5R; 10S	5R; 10S	5R; 10S
			3R; 5S	3R; 5S

STRETCHING PROGRAM—LEVEL 2

	WEEK		
	1	2	3
Head Turns (L1)	5R; 3S	10R; 5S	10R; 5S
Chin to Chest (L1)	5R; 3S	5R; 5S	5R; 5S
Front Arm Raises (L1)	8R; 1S		
Side Arm Raises (L1)	8R; 1S		
Shoulder Stretches (L1)	5R; 3S		
Side Leans (L1)	3R; 5S	5R; 8S	5R; 8S
Knee Touches (L1)	5R; 8S	5R; 10S	5R; 10S
Seated Toe Touches (L1)	3R; 5S	3R; 5S	3R; 5S
Shoulder Rolls (L2)		5R	10R
Alternate Arm across Chest (L2)		5R; 3S	5R; 3S
Front Arm Circles (L2)		10R	10R
Side Arm Circles (L2)		10R	10R
Knees to Chest (L2)			3R; 5S
Head Tilts (L2)			
Advanced Seated Toe Touches (L3)			
Quadriceps Stretches (L3)			
Wall Leans (L3)			
Triceps Stretches (L3)			
Butterflies (L3)			

R=repetitions; S=time to hold stretch (sec)

4	5	6	7	8
10R; 5S	10R; 5S	10R; 5S	10R; 5S	10R; 5S
5R; 5S	5R; 5S	5R; 5S	5R; 5S	5R; 5S
5R; 8S	5R; 8S	5R; 8S	5R; 8S	5R; 8S
10R	15R	15R	15R	15R
5R; 3S	5R; 3S	5R; 5S	5R; 5S	5R; 5S
10R	15R	15R	15R	15R
10R	15R	15R	15R	15R
3R; 5S	5R; 5S	5R; 5S	5R; 5S	5R; 5S
3R; 5S	3R; 5S	5R; 5S	5R; 5S	5R; 5S
5R; 10S	5R; 10S	5R; 10S	5R; 10S	5R; 10S
	3R; 5S	3R; 5S	3R; 8S	3R; 8S
	2R; 5S	2R; 5S	3R; 5S	3R; 5S
	5R; 10S	5R; 10S	5R; 10S	5R; 10S
		3R; 5S	3R; 5S	3R; 5S

STRETCHING PROGRAM—LEVEL 3

	WEEK		
	1	2	3
Head Turns (L1)	5R; 3S	10R; 5S	10R; 5S
Chin to Chest (L1)	5R; 3S	5R; 5S	5R; 5S
Side Leans (L1)	3R; 5S	5R; 8S	5R; 8S
Knee Touches (L1)	5R; 10S		
Seated Toe Touches (L1)	3R; 5S		
Shoulder Rolls (L2)	5R	8R	10R
Alternate Arm across Chest (L2)	5R; 3S	5R; 3S	5R; 3S
Front Arm Circles (L2)	10R	10R	15R
Side Arm Circles (L2)	10R	10R	15R
Knees to Chest (L2)			3R; 5S
Head Tilts (L3)		3R; 5S	3R; 5S
Advanced Seated Toe Touches (L3)		3R; 5S	3R; 10S
Quadriceps Stretches (L3)			
Wall Leans (L3)			
Triceps Stretches (L3)			
Butterflies (L3)			

R=repetitions; S=time to hold stretch (sec)

to the floor, hold, then slowly lower them back to the starting position. Repeat as indicated.

Shoulder Stretches: Stand straight with your arms at your sides. Raise your right arm, reach across your chest, and touch the top of your

4	5	6	7	8
10R; 5S	10R; 5S	10R; 5S	10R; 5S	10R; 5S
5R; 5S	5R; 5S	5R; 5S	5R; 5S	5R; 5S
5R; 8S	5R; 8S	5R; 8S	5R; 8S	5R; 8S
10R	15R	15R	15R	15R
5R; 3S	5R; 3S	5R; 5S	5R; 5S	5R; 5S
15R	15R	15R	15R	15R
15R	15R	15R	15R	15R
3R; 5S	5R; 5S	5R; 5S	5R; 5S	5R; 5S
5R; 5S	5R; 5S	5R; 5S	5R; 5S	5R; 5S
5R; 10S	5R; 10S	5R; 10S	5R; 10S	5R; 10S
3R; 5S	3R; 5S	3R; 8S	3R; 8S	3R; 8S
2R; 5S	2R; 5S	3R; 5S	3R; 5S	3R; 5S
5R; 10S	5R; 10S	5R; 10S	5R; 10S	5R; 10S
3R; 5S	3R; 5S	3R; 5S	3R; 10S	3R; 10S

left shoulder with your hand. Place your left hand on your right elbow, then slowly reach with your right hand over your left shoulder toward your back. Your right elbow should be bent as if you were reaching for your shoulder blade, with your left hand just supporting it; do not push on your elbow to extend the stretch. Hold, then relax the tension before repeating. Repeat as indicated, then repeat with your left arm.

Side Leans: Stand straight with your arms at your sides. Slowly lean to the left, reaching down toward the outside of your left foot. (As you lean, imagine a flat surface, such as a sheet of plywood, running through the middle of your body and lean parallel to that plane—don't bend forward or backward.) Hold, then slowly return to the starting position. Repeat as indicated, then repeat on the right side.

Knee Touches: Sit in a straight-backed chair and place your right leg on the seat of another chair so that your leg is almost parallel to the floor (or sit on the floor with your legs extended in front of you). Slowly reach down with both hands and touch your right knee, then slide your hands toward your foot until you feel a slight tension, but don't force the stretch. Hold, then relax the tension before repeating as indicated. Repeat with your left leg.

Seated Toe Touches: Sit upright in a straight-backed chair with both feet squarely on the floor. Slowly lean over and touch your toes (because your knees are bent at a right angle, your arms will pass beside your knees, not over them). Hold, then slowly return to the starting position and rest for 5 seconds before repeating as indicated.

L2 Stretches

Shoulder Rolls: Stand straight with your arms at your sides. Simultaneously roll both shoulders back for the specified number of repetitions, then roll them forward.

Alternate Arm across Chest (replaces L1 Shoulder Stretch): Stand straight with your arms at your sides. Raise your right arm and extend it across your chest and past your left arm, so that your right elbow is in front of your upper chest. Place your left hand on your right forearm and pull your right arm toward your chest. Hold, then release the tension before repeating as indicated. Repeat with your left arm.

Front Arm Circles (replaces L1 Front Arm Raise): Stand straight with your arms at your sides. Slowly raise them simultaneously in front of you until they are parallel to the floor, then rotate them inward (toward each other) in circles about 6 to 12 inches in diameter. Repeat as indicated, then rotate your arms outward.

Side Arm Circles (replaces L1 Side Arm Raise): Stand straight with your arms at your sides. Slowly raise them simultaneously out to the sides until they are parallel to the floor, then rotate them forward in circles about 6 to 12 inches in diameter. Repeat as indicated, then rotate your arms backward.

Knees to Chest: Lie on your back on a firm but comfortable surface with your knees bent and your feet flat on the floor. Place your hands behind your knees and raise them toward your chest. Hold, then slowly return to the starting position. Repeat as indicated.

L3 Stretches

Head Tilts: Sit or stand with your head erect and facing forward. Relax your shoulders and slowly tilt your head toward your left shoulder, hold, then slowly raise it and tilt it toward your right shoulder. Don't dip your head forward or backward as you tilt it. Repeat as indicated.

Advanced Seated Toe Touches (replaces L1 Seated Toe Touches and Knee Touches): Sit on a firm but comfortable surface with your legs extended and your knees slightly bent. Slowly reach out to touch your toes. Hold, then slowly return to the starting position. Repeat as indicated.

Quadriceps Stretches: Stand behind a straight-backed chair and hold on to the back with your right hand to balance yourself. Bend your left knee and raise your leg toward your buttocks. Grasp your ankle or pants leg with your left hand and gently pull your leg closer to your buttocks until you feel the stretch, then hold. Slowly lower your leg to the starting position. Repeat as indicated, then use your left hand for balance and repeat with your right leg.

Wall Leans: Stand facing a wall and about a foot away from it. Bend your elbows and place both hands on the wall about shoulder-width apart. Keeping your heels on the floor, slowly slide your feet backward in small increments until they are back as far as they can go comfortably and without strain—about 2 to 3 feet from the wall. Be sure that your heels are still flat on the floor. To increase the stretch, keep your feet flat on the floor and slowly lean a few inches toward the wall. (You should move your feet only far enough to feel a gentle stretch when you lean into the wall, but not so far that you feel as if you are doing a pushup against the wall.) You should feel a slight stretch in your calves, but not tight pulling or pain. Hold, then relax, push away from the wall, and repeat as indicated.

Triceps Stretches: Sit or stand with your head erect and facing forward. Reach up with your right arm and place your hand behind your neck, between your shoulder blades. Place your left hand on your right elbow and gently push it up and back. Hold, then release the tension. Repeat as indicated, then repeat with your left arm.

Butterflies: Sit on a firm but comfortable surface with your knees bent and the soles of your feet together. Grasp your feet with both hands and bring them toward your body as far as possible while keeping your knees comfortably bent. Lean your upper body forward toward your feet until you feel a slight stretch in your groin muscles. Hold, then relax for 15 seconds. Repeat as indicated.

MAINTENANCE

When you have finished your 8-Week Stretching Program, repeat the sit-and–reach test in chapter 4 and move to the next level as appropriate. When you complete the Level 3 program, you may continue at that level with these stretches, or you may wish to explore a wider range of stretches. Check the recommended books in the Resources for more information.

STRONG MUSCLES FOR JOINT HEALTH

Properly conditioned and toned muscles are critically important to joint health. As noted in chapter 2, the interaction of joints and muscles is complex. Often, muscle weakness is the underlying cause of a joint injury. Think, for example, of the weekend warrior who does nothing to condition his muscles during the week, then plays tennis on Saturday and tears cartilage in his knee. In most instances, participating in regular strength training can make the joints more stable and help prevent this type of injury. In addition, strength training can help people who have joint problems achieve significantly improved function and decreased pain. Of equal importance, maintaining strong, flexible muscles can significantly lower your risk of developing joint problems in later years.

BENEFITS OF MUSCLE FUNCTION AND STRENGTH

Properly conditioned muscles play at least four major roles in maintaining or enhancing joint health.

Movement. Joints enable our bodies to move and interact with the environment. Without muscles, however, joints would have only the potential to move, because the muscles that cross over each joint generate the force that allows movement. By contracting and relaxing in coordinated sets, our muscles put our joints through all the possible permutations of movement. Weak muscles limit movement and control of movement. Stronger muscles enable assured, precise movement.

Joint stability. Safe movement for both your joints and your whole body requires stable joints. Joint stability, both when our bodies are in motion and when they are at rest, requires strong muscles. Although the ligaments that connect the bones that meet in the joint provide stability, they depend on strong muscles to prevent excessive motion (such as hyperextension), which can stretch and damage the ligaments. One of the problems that injured athletes experience is that their muscles become weak, possibly undermining joint stability. That's why strength training is such an important part of rehabilitation for injuries (including the damage or injury from osteoarthritis). More important, strengthening your muscles and keeping them strong reinforces joint stability and decreases the likelihood of injury in the first place.

Shock absorption. Muscles also help a joint absorb shock. In fact, although the analogy is not perfect, you can compare them to the shock absorbers in your car. The shock absorbers are not the joints that connect the car's wheels to the axle and body of the car, but they support and buffer those joints. When you drive your car over a railroad track, the wheels rattle up and down, but the body of the car and its occupants enjoy a much smoother ride.

Now imagine that you are riding a bicycle. Do you stay seated as you approach the track? Not on your life! Without even thinking about it, you rise on the pedals. As the bicycle bumps across the track, your legs, feet, hands, and arms all flex swiftly and gracefully up and down, dissipating the impact and sparing your joints, spine, and especially your head from an awful jarring. The mechanisms that allow your limbs and joints to move so efficiently to absorb the shock are your muscles. Although this scenario's a bit extreme, it shows you in large terms the role that your muscles play in every step you take and every move you make.

Because weak muscles simply cannot carry out adequate shock absorption, the result is increased stress on the joints and increased potential for wear and tear and injury.

Sensory functions. Muscles also play a very important sensory role. They are connected to the nervous system in ways that allow constant feedback to the brain about the position of the joints. If the muscles are weak and therefore poorly aligned, it is possible that the joint will also be poorly aligned, setting up a higher potential for injury. Think of what happens when the stairs end one step before you think they do, and your misinformed muscles don't react properly. Some bone-jarring impact, right? Muscles that are well-conditioned send better signals about joint position to your brain, allowing you to achieve a more aligned and coordinated gait when walking or climbing stairs, for instance. Strong muscles are also better able to recover and protect your joints at those moments when your preoccupied brain sends out the wrong instructions about those stairs or some other obstacle.

OTHER HEALTH BENEFITS

Beyond their specific contributions to joint function, muscles provide other benefits for joint health. For instance, strong muscles help maintain or increase functional fitness as we age. They also promote increased bone density and slow the damage of osteoporosis. Because strength training is the only real way to increase lean muscle mass, and because more lean muscle burns more calories (increases your metabolism), stronger muscles also help in lifelong weight control.

IT'S NEVER TOO EARLY OR TOO LATE TO START

Even if you currently have no joint problems, and whatever your age, strength training for joint health is very important. In fact, one of the best times to do strength training is when your muscles and joints do not need to overcome injuries in order to benefit from it. People who have not previously done strength training can often experience a 50 to 100 percent increase in strength by doing it regularly. This can make a big difference in joint health and help with the factors that I have already mentioned to decrease the likelihood of joint problems.

WHAT IF YOU ALREADY HAVE JOINT PROBLEMS?

As I mentioned, strength training is a key component of rehabilitation for people who are injured or have chronic joint problems. Those who have osteoarthritis in their hips or knees often experience significant decreases in muscle strength, but, as a number of research studies have shown, regular strength training can increase the functional abilities of their joints by 30 to 50 percent and can also decrease pain to a similar extent. Of course, if you have existing problems, it is very important to consult a physician or a physical therapist who can develop specific strength-training programs to help rehabilitate any joint that you are having problems with. The 8-Week Strength-Training Program is generally safe for people with a wide range of abilities, but you will want to consult a health professional to adapt them to your needs and limitations.

THE 8-WEEK STRENGTH-TRAINING PROGRAM

These strength-training programs have been designed especially for people who want to work toward healthy, pain-free joints. You should select the program that's right for you, based on the results that you achieved on the Joint Health Index and the strength test in chapter 4 and recorded on your Joint Health Profile Card.

If you have pain or problem in any joint, you should consult your physician before starting this program. These routines, however, have been designed to be safe for people who may have mild osteoarthritis.

EQUIPMENT

- Comfortable clothing suitable for exercise
- Comfortable cross-training or walking shoes with nonslip soles (don't lift in your loafers)
- Two straight-backed chairs, such as dining chairs that don't roll
- One straight-backed chair with arms
- Ankle weights adjustable to 10 or 15 pounds (these are inexpensive and available at sporting goods stores)
- Dumbbells—2, 4, 5, 6, 8, 10, 12, and 15 pounds (or adjustable to 15 pounds)

GENERAL GUIDELINES

1. Always do a warmup and cooldown; include light stretching in both.
2. Try to breathe normally as you perform each exercise. Holding your breath makes your heart work harder and can be dangerous to your cardiovascular system. Instead, use your breathing to enhance your efficiency by breathing in rhythm with your lifting—exhale as you contract the muscle and inhale as you release the lift.
3. Always allow a day of rest for your muscles between strength workouts. That means that you should either do strength training every other day or do lower-body exercises and upper-body exercises on alternate days.

THE STRENGTH-TRAINING EXERCISES

The purpose of this program is to build strong muscles and increase functional fitness as safely as possible while allowing you to make real progress. As in the stretching programs, the individual exercises within the program for each level are designated as L1, L2, or L3. Thus, although your test scores place you in Level 1, for example, that level's program includes some L2 and L3 exercises. Again, as you progress through the program, you will continue to do some exercises, while you will replace others with higher-level ones.

Each level starts slowly and builds up progressively, increasing the intensity of the workouts at a cautious but consistent pace. Patience, in this case, is a virtue that will pay off. If you are accustomed to thinking of strength training as weight training, when looking at the first weeks of training sessions, you may wonder where the weight is. At the beginning of the program, your body serves as the weight that your muscles "lift" or "resist."

In each session, perform all the exercises in the order given. The chart for each level indicates how many repetitions and sets—groups of repetitions—you should do for each exercise. When the instructions specify doing an exercise with one arm or leg and then the other, you should begin by changing sides after each set, which gives the muscles a chance to recover between sets. When you want a little more challenge, you may do all the sets for one side and then the sets for the other side. When you do this or do exercises that work both sides of the body together, rest for at least 15 seconds, but no more than a minute, between sets.

L1 Exercises (Lower-Body Routine)

Seated Lower-Leg Extensions: Sit in a straight-backed chair with your feet flat on the floor. Slowly raise your right leg so that it is parallel to the floor, then slowly return to the starting position. Repeat as indicated, then repeat with your left leg.

Seated Toe Raises: Sit in a straight-backed chair with your feet flat on the floor. Slowly lift your feet so that only your toes touch the floor, then slowly return to the starting position. Repeat as indicated.

L2 Exercises (Lower-Body Routine)

Lying Leg Curls: Lie flat on your stomach on a firm but comfortable surface. Slowly curl (bend) both legs up toward your buttocks, then slowly lower them to the floor. Repeat as indicated.

Outer-Leg Lifts: Lie on your left side on a firm but comfortable surface with your legs extended. Support yourself with your left arm and slowly lift your right leg vertically in a scissors-like motion. Slowly return to the starting position. Repeat as indicated, then lie on your right side and repeat with your left leg.

Weighted Leg Extensions (replaces L1 Seated Lower-Leg Extensions): Sit in a straight-backed chair with your feet on the floor and attach the specified ankle weights. Slowly raise your right leg parallel to the floor, then slowly lower it. Repeat as indicated, then repeat with your left leg.

Standing Toe Raises (replaces L1 Seated Toe Raises): Stand behind a straight-backed chair and hold on to the back with both hands for balance. Start with your feet flat on the floor, slowly rise up on your toes, then slowly return to the starting position. Repeat as indicated.

L3 Exercises (Lower-Body Routine)

Inner-Leg Lifts: Lie on your left side on a firm but comfortable surface with your legs extended. Use your left arm to support yourself and move your right leg slightly behind the left so that your right foot is touching the floor. Slowly raise your left leg vertically in a scissors-like motion, then slowly lower it. Repeat as indicated, then lie on your right side and repeat with your right leg.

STRENGTH-TRAINING PROGRAM—LEVEL 1

	WEEK		
	1	2	3
LOWER-BODY EXERCISES			
Seated Lower-Leg Extensions (L1)	10R; 2S; 0#	15R; 3S; 0#	20R; 4S; 0#
Seated Toe Raises (L1)	10R; 2S; 0#	15R; 3S; 0#	20R; 4S 0#
Lying Leg Curls (L2)			
Outer-Leg Lifts (L2)			
Weighted Leg Extensions (L2)			
Standing Toe Raises (L2)			
Inner-Leg Lifts (L3)			
Weighted Leg Curls (L3)			
Chair Squats (L3)			
UPPER-BODY EXERCISES			
Chin Crunches (L1)	10R; 2S 0#	15R; 3S; 0#	20R; 4S; 0#
Triceps Extensions (L1)	10R; 3S; 0#	15R; 3S; 0#	20R; 4S; 0#
Seated Biceps Curls (L1)	10R; 3S; 0#	15R; 3S; 0#	20R; 4S; 0#
Abdominal Crunches (L2)			
Dumbbell Triceps Kickbacks (L2)			
Dumbbell Shoulder Presses (L3)			
Dumbbell Chest Presses (L3)			

R=repetitions; S=sets; #=weight (lb)

Weighted Leg Curls (replaces L2 Lying Leg Curls): Attach the specified ankle weights, then lie flat on your stomach on a firm but comfortable surface. Slowly curl (bend) both legs up toward your buttocks, then slowly lower them. Repeat as indicated.

	4	5	6	7	8
	10R; 2S; 0#	10R; 3S; 0#	15R; 3S; 0#		
	5R; 2;S; 0#	10R; 2S; 0#	10R; 3S; 0#	10R; 3S; 2#	15R; 3S; 2#
	10R; 3S; 2#	15R; 3S; 2#	20R; 3S; 2#	15R; 3S; 4#	20R; 3S; 4#
	10R; 3S; 0#	15R; 3S; 0#	20R; 3S; 0#	25R; 3S; 0#	30R; 3S; 0#
				5R; 2S; 0#	10R; 2S; 0#
				10R; 3S; 2#	15R; 3S; 4#
				3R; 2S; 0#	5R; 3S; 0#
	15R; 3S; 2#	15R; 3S; 4#	15R; 3S; 6#	15R; 3S; 8#	15R; 3S; 10#
	10R; 2S; 0#	15R; 3S; 0#	20R; 3S; 0#	25R; 3S; 0#	30R; 3S; 0#
	15R; 3S; 2#	15R; 3S; 4#	15R; 3S; 5#	20R; 3S; 5#	15R; 3S; 6#
				10R; 3S; 2#	15R; 3S; 2#
				10R; 3S; 2#	15R; 3S; 2#

Chair Squats: Sit at the edge of a straight-backed chair with your feet flat on the floor in front of you and shoulder-width apart, with your toes pointed slightly outward. Extend your arms in front of you for balance and slowly stand up, keeping your back straight. Then, keep your

STRENGTH-TRAINING PROGRAM—LEVEL 2

	WEEK		
	1	2	3
LOWER-BODY EXERCISES			
Lying Leg Curls (L2)	10R; 2S; 0#	10R; 3S; 0#	15R; 3S; 0#
Outer-Leg Lifts (L2)	5R; 2S; 0#	10R; 2S; 0#	10R; 3S; 0#
Weighted Leg Extensions (L2)	10R; 3S; 2#	15R; 3S; 2#	20R; 3S; 2#
Standing Toe Raises (L2)	10R; 3S; 0#	15R; 3S; 0#	20R; 3S; 0#
Inner-Leg Lifts (L3)			
Weighted Leg Curls (L3)			
Chair Squats (L3)			
UPPER-BODY EXERCISES			
Seated Biceps Curls (L1)	15R; 3S; 2#	15R; 3S; 4#	15R; 3S; 6#
Abdominal Crunches (L2)	10R; 2S; 0#	15R; 3S; 0#	20R; 3S; 0#
Dumbbell Triceps Kickbacks (L2)	15R; 3S; 2#	15R; 3S; 4#	15R; 3S; 5#
Dumbbell Shoulder Presses (L3)			
Dumbbell Chest Presses (L3)			

R=repetitions; S=sets; #=weight (lb)

head facing forward, move backward slightly, and lower yourself until your buttocks touch the chair. (Be sure that your knees never extend past your toes when you stand up, and keep your feet flat on the floor throughout the exercise.) Repeat as indicated.

L1 Exercises (Upper-Body Routine)

Chin Crunches: Lie flat on your back on a firm but comfortable surface with a rolled towel under your head. Keep your arms

	4	5	6	7	8
	10R; 3S; 2#	15R; 3S; 2#	10R; 3S; 4#	15R; 3S; 4#	15R; 3S; 6#
	15R; 3S; 4#	20R; 3S; 4#	15R; 3S; 6#	15R; 3S; 8#	15R; 3S; 10#
	25R; 3S; 0#	30R; 3S; 0#	30R; 3S; 0#	30R; 3S; 0#	30R; 3S; 0#
	5R; 2S; 0#	10R; 2S; 0#	8R; 3S; 0#	10R; 3S; 0#	12R; 3S; 0#
	10R; 3S; 2#	15R; 3S; 4#	20R; 3S; 4#	15R; 3S; 6#	20R; 3S; 6#
	3R; 2S; 0#	5R; 3S; 0#	8R; 3S; 0#	10R; 3S; 0#	12R; 3S; 0#
	15R; 3S; 8#	15R; 3S; 10#	15R; 3S; 10#	15R; 3S; 12#	15R; 3S; 15#
	25R; 3S; 0#	30R; 3S; 0#	35R; 3S; 0#	35R; 3S; 0#	40R; 3S; 0#
	20R; 3S; 5#	15R; 3S; 6#	20R; 3S; 6#	15R; 3S; 8#	20R; 3S; 8#
		10R; 3S; 2#	15R; 3S; 2#	10R; 3S; 5#	15R; 3S; 5#
		10R; 3S; 2#	15R; 3S; 2#	10R; 3S; 5#	15R; 3S; 5#

at your sides and slowly raise your chin toward your chest. Hold for the specified amount of time, then lower your head. Repeat as indicated.

Seated Biceps Curls: Sit in a straight-backed chair with your arms at your sides. Slowly raise your right hand and touch your right shoulder, then slowly lower it to the starting position. Repeat with your left arm, then continue to alternate arms for the specified number of repetitions per set.

STRENGTH-TRAINING PROGRAM—LEVEL 3

	WEEK		
	1	2	3
LOWER-BODY EXERCISES			
Outer-Leg Lifts (L2)	5R; 3S; 0#	10R; 3S; 0#	10R; 3S; 2#
Weighted Leg Extensions (L2)	10R; 2S; 5#	10R; 3S; 5#	15R; 3S; 5#
Standing Toe Raises (L2)	10R; 3S; 0#	15R; 3S; 0#	20R; 3S; 0#
Inner-Leg Lifts (L3)			5R; 3S; 0#
Weighted Leg Curls (L3)			10R; 3S; 2#
Chair Squats (L3)			3R; 2S; 0#
UPPER-BODY EXERCISES			
Seated Biceps Curls (L1)	15R; 3S; 5#	15R; 3S; 8#	15R; 3S; 10#
Abdominal Crunches (L2)	10R; 3S; 0#	15R; 3S; 0#	20R; 3S; 0#
Dumbbell Triceps Kickbacks (L2)	10R; 3S; 5#	15R; 3S; 5#	20R; 3S; 5#
Dumbbell Shoulder Presses (L3)		10R; 3S; 5#	15R; 3S; 5#
Dumbbell Chest Presses (L3)		10R; 3S; 5#	15R; 3S; 5#

R=repetitions; S=sets; # = weight (lb)

Triceps Extensions: Sit in a straight-backed chair and move your right hand across your chest so that it touches the top of your left shoulder. Place your left hand under your right elbow for support, straighten your right arm so that it is parallel to the floor, then return to the starting position. Repeat as indicated, then repeat with your left arm.

L2 Exercises (Upper-Body Routine)

Abdominal Crunches (replaces L1 Chin Crunches): Lie flat on your back on a firm but comfortable surface and place your lower legs on the seat of a chair so that your knees are bent at the edge of the seat.

4	5	6	7	8
10R; 3S; 5#	15R; 3S; 5#	20R; 3S; 5#	20R; 3S; 7#	15R; 3S; 10#
15R; 3S; 8#	15R; 3S; 10#	15R; 3S; 10#	15R; 3S; 12#	15R; 3S; 12#
25R; 3S; 0#	30R; 3S; 0#	30R; 3S; 0#	35R; 3S; 0#	35R; 3S; 0#
10R; 3S; 0#	15R; 3S; 0#	15R; 3S; 2#	15R; 3S; 4#	15R; 3S; 6#
15R; 3S; 4#	20R; 3S; 4#	15R; 3S; 6#	20R; 3S; 6#	15R; 3S; 8#
5R; 3S; 0#	8R; 3S; 0#	10R; 3S; 0#	15R; 3S; 0#	20R; 3S; 0#
15R; 3S; 15#	15R; 3S; 15#	20R; 3S; 15#	10R; 3S; 20#	15R; 3S; 20#
25R; 3S; 0#	30R; 3S; 0#	35R; 3S; 0#	40R; 3S; 0#	45R; 3S; 0#
15R; 3S; 8#	20R; 3S; 8#	15R; 3S; 10#	20R; 3S; 10#	15R; 3S; 15#
10R; 3S; 8#	15R; 3S; 8#	10R; 3S; 10#	15R; 3S; 10#	15R; 3S; 15#
10R; 3S; 8#	15R; 3S; 8#	10R; 3S; 10#	15R; 3S; 10#	15R; 3S; 15#

Cross your arms over your chest. Using your abdominal muscles, curl (roll up) toward your knees, raising your shoulders about 3 inches. Hold, then return to the starting position. Repeat as indicated.

Dumbbell Triceps Kickbacks (replaces L1 Triceps Extensions): Stand facing a chair with armrests. Place your right hand on the left armrest and your right knee on the seat near the armrest so that you are leaning at a slight 45-degree angle and looking over the back of the chair. Hold a dumbbell of the specified weight in your left hand and let your arm hang by your side, with your elbow close to your body. (During the exercise, your upper arm should stay parallel to your body;

only your elbow should bend.) Slowly lift the weight toward your left shoulder, then extend your forearm down and behind you until your elbow is fully extended but not hyperextended. Repeat as indicated, then put your left knee on the chair, hold on to the right armrest with your left hand, and repeat with your right arm.

L3 Exercises (Upper-Body Routine)

Dumbbell Shoulder Presses: Sit in a straight-backed chair with a dumbbell of the specified weight in each hand. Lift both weights toward your shoulders, with your elbows bent and your palms facing away from you. Straighten your left arm and raise the weight above your shoulder, then lower it to the starting position. Repeat with your right arm, then continue to alternate arms for the specified number of repetitions per set.

Dumbbell Chest Presses: Lie on your back on a firm but comfortable surface with a dumbbell of the specified weight in each hand. Lift both weights toward your shoulders, with your elbows bent and your palms facing away from you. Straighten your left arm and lift the weight straight up above your shoulder, then lower it to the starting position. Repeat with your right arm, then continue to alternate arms for the specified number of repetitions per set.

MAINTENANCE

When you finish your first 8-week program, retake the strength test in chapter 4 and assess your progress. You'll probably be ready to move up a level. When you have completed Level 3, you can maintain a good functional level of strength by using this program as a regular routine.

If you enjoy the results of your strength-training program as much as I think you will, you may wish to pursue it further. You may want to work out at a health club with a strength-training specialist or explore more options in home-based strength training. To learn more, check the Resources.

DEXTERITY FOR HANDS AND FINGERS

The joints of your hands and fingers present special challenges when it comes to exercise. Many people experience the pain and stiffness of osteoarthritis more in their hands than in any other joints. Because our hands are busy all day long, it would seem that they get plenty of physical activity, but actually, pain and stiffness can cause us to use them less or limit the range of motion.

The following dexterity exercises can help keep your hand and finger joints pain-free and functioning at a high level, either before problems start or if you have mild osteoarthritis symptoms. The exercises won't be the most fascinating thing you do every day, but think of them as 10 finger exercises for an active life.

Start at the level indicated by your tests in chapter 4. Do the exercises daily, and when you feel you are ready, add exercises from the next level. I recommend that you make these exercises part of your stretching routine, but you can also tuck them into the nooks and crannies of the day. Doing a few while you watch your favorite show or sporting event on TV (at least during the commercials) is a great way to work them in.

THE 8-WEEK DEXTERITY PROGRAM

Level 1

Finger-to-Thumb Touch: Hold your right hand out in front of you with the palm up. Slowly move each finger in sequence to touch your thumb, starting with your index finger and ending with your pinky finger. Then work backward, from your pinky to your index finger. Speed up your movements and continue for 30 seconds, then do the exercise with your left hand. As your hands grow more flexible over the weeks of your program, the number of reps you can do in 30 seconds will gradually increase.

Level 2

Finger Stretch: Sit at a table and rest your hands on the tabletop. Make fists with both hands, then simultaneously extend your fingers and thumbs as far as possible. Hold for 1 second, then return to the starting position. Repeat 10 times, then rest for 30 seconds. Start with three sets and add another set every 2 weeks.

Wrist Roll: Find an 18-inch-long stick or pipe that you can easily hold in your hands. Tie a piece of rope or string at least 3 feet long in the middle so that the string hangs to the floor when you stand up. Hold the stick in both hands and use your wrists to roll it so that the string wraps around it, then roll it down to the floor again. This is 1 repetition. Start with 5 repetitions, resting for 10 seconds after each. Add 1 repetition each week until you reach 8 to 10.

Level 3

Advanced Finger-to-Thumb Touch: Stand erect with your arms at your sides. Hold both hands in front of you with the palms up, face forward, and do the finger-to-thumb touch with both hands simultaneously. Speed up your movements and continue for 30 seconds.

Crumple: Hold a small towel in your left hand. Using only that hand, crumple the towel so that it is completely within your hand. Then repeat with your right hand. Start by doing 5 repetitions with each hand and build up to at least 10, adding 1 a week.

MAINTENANCE

Continue doing your dexterity exercises daily.

Managing Your Weight

Let me be blunt. Our nation has become too fat, and every aspect of our health is suffering because of it. When it comes to joint health, the facts about obesity are very stark. Obesity is the number one cause of osteoarthritis in women in the United States and the number two cause (behind previous injuries) of osteoarthritis in men. If you want to keep your joints healthy for life, one of the very best decisions that you can make is to maintain a proper weight throughout your life. Even if you already have joint disease and are overweight, one of the most beneficial things that you can do is to lose weight to take some of the stress off your weight-bearing joints, such as your knees, ankles, and hips.

The adverse effects of obesity go far beyond the negative impact on joint health. In fact, obesity and its associated conditions are the second leading cause of preventable deaths in the United States (second only to cigarette smoking), resulting in more than 300,000 deaths each year. If obesity continues to increase at the current rate in our country, sometime in the next decade, it will surpass cigarette smoking as the leading cause of preventable deaths.

The extent and growth of this obesity epidemic are truly shocking. In the past decade, the prevalence of obesity in the United States has increased by 40 percent. Depending on the criteria used, between 25 and 35 percent of the adult population is now clinically obese, and more than half of the adult population is at least somewhat overweight. Unfortunately, this epidemic extends to children as well. The prevalence of obesity among children in this country has doubled in the past 20 years. So, if you are overweight and thinking about losing a few pounds to give your joints some relief, think also about helping your children or grandchildren maintain proper weight. This is one of the best things that they can do to maintain overall good health as well as healthy joints throughout their lives.

In an otherwise bleak picture, the good news is that losing weight—even as little as 10 pounds—and maintaining that loss can have a positive effect on your joint health as well as your overall health.

First, let's look further at the link between weight and joint health. Then I'll give you some guidance about the most effective ways to lose weight if you are overweight or maintain a healthy weight if you are not.

HOW MUCH WEIGHT IS TOO MUCH?

If your body mass index (BMI) places you in one of the categories defined as overweight or obese, you are jeopardizing your joints. As explained in chapter 4, scientific studies use BMI because it very accurately reflects an individual's level of body fat. Anyone whose BMI is greater than 25 is considered overweight, and anyone with a BMI of 30 or greater is considered obese.

A lot of us consider ourselves to be at an average weight or a little overweight, and we think of obesity as something that occurs in others. A quick look at the BMI chart on page 50, however, will show that it doesn't take many extra pounds to become overweight or obese. Take the average 5'10" man in the United States, for example. At 175 pounds, he is technically overweight; at 201, he would be considered obese. An average 5'4" woman who weighs 146 pounds is considered overweight. If she added another 30 pounds to reach 176, she would be considered obese. And unfortunately, those extra pounds tend to sneak up on us over the years. The average adult gains 1 pound each year after the age of 20.

So, if you wonder whether you are overweight or obese, simply look at your Joint Health Profile Card to see what your BMI is (or turn back to chapter 4 to determine it). If you have a BMI over 25, the yellow caution flag should come out, and you should strongly consider losing weight, not only for joint health but also for general health. If your BMI is greater than 30, you certainly have a very significant risk factor for problems with your joints as well as other adverse effects on your health.

THE EFFECT ON YOUR JOINTS

Too many pounds, studies show, damage primarily the knee joints. Damage occurs first because extra weight increases the pounding that the cartilage and all other structures in the joint take as you walk, climb stairs, sit and rise, and just carry out everyday activities. Other more complicated, interrelated factors also appear to play a role, however. For instance, people who are significantly overweight have difficulty achieving proper alignment of their knees. This misalignment can further exacerbate joint problems, and as these problems make physical activity more uncomfortable, overweight people become less active. Reduced physical activity in turn produces weaker muscles and joint structures. The joints then suffer not only from the increased pounding of the excess weight but also from the decreased ability of the muscles and ligaments to cushion that impact. As you see, these events set up a vicious cycle. The longer that cycle continues and the more momentum it gathers, the more rapidly joints decline, leading to major joint problems and perhaps costly surgery.

In some cases, being only a few pounds overweight too early or for too long can have adverse effects. A major study from Johns Hopkins University, for example, showed that people with a BMI of 25 or greater (think of the 5'10" man who weighs 175 pounds or the 5'4" woman who weighs 146 pounds) who carried this extra weight in their twenties had a threefold increase in the likelihood of arthritis in their knees by the time they reached their sixties.

LOWERING YOUR RISK OF JOINT PROBLEMS

Fortunately, a little loss can result in a big gain for your joints. Data from the Framingham Osteoarthritis Study showed that women who were overweight and who lost an average of 10 pounds decreased their likelihood of developing osteoarthritis of the knee by 50 percent.

Losing Excess Weight Benefits Your Total Health

Although this chapter focuses on how weight affects your joints, it is important to remember that being overweight or obese also has multiple negative consequences for your general health. It increases risks for the following conditions and also causes these risk factors to cluster in groups of two, three, or more.

▓ Heart disease
▓ High blood pressure (contributes to 40 to 70 percent of high blood pressure)
▓ High cholesterol (is associated with over half of all lipid, or fat, problems)
▓ Diabetes (accounts for 85 percent of type 2, or non-insulin-dependent, diabetes)
▓ Certain cancers
▓ Depression

The good news is that studies have shown that even more than in joint health, losing 5 to 10 percent of total body weight results in a significant decrease in risk factors for heart disease and other chronic diseases. Thus, you don't have to reach your optimal weight to achieve a healthier weight.

As you can imagine, if you already have joint problems, anything that reduces the stress and impact on your joints will be beneficial. Therefore, weight loss in people who have existing osteoarthritis of the knee or hip can help decrease symptoms and increase function. Nothing is truer for your joint health than that old saying, "every little bit helps."

THE BEST WAY TO LOSE WEIGHT

Over the past 25 years, thousands of researchers in hundreds of studies have examined the mechanisms of how people gain weight and the most effective ways to lose it. The findings are remarkably consistent, simple, and easy to understand.

▓ Consuming more calories than the body burns produces weight gain.
▓ Conversely, burning more calories than the body consumes produces weight loss.

Of course, a number of personal, social, and psychological factors may play a role in why someone consumes more calories than she burns or finds it difficult to burn more calories than she consumes in order to lose weight, but physiologically, those are the mechanisms.

Given this physiological reality, there are basically three different ways to lose weight.

- Cutting down on the number of calories taken in—dieting
- Increasing the number of calories burned—exercise
- Combining fewer calories consumed with more calories burned— dieting combined with increased exercise and physical activity

Here is a summary of the effectiveness of each of these approaches.

Dieting. Extensive research shows that the most effective way to lose a significant amount of weight in the short term is to restrict the number of calories that you take in. That's why most effective weight-loss diet plans restrict calories to create a calorie deficit of at least 500 calories per day. While calorie restriction works as a short-term solution and is absolutely vital to a weight-loss program, most people find that if they do not make other fundamental changes in their lives—in particular, increasing their physical activity or exercise—it is very hard to keep weight off long-term.

Increasing exercise/physical activity. Although increased exercise or physical activity is vitally important in maintaining weight loss, most studies have shown that simply increasing exercise while consuming the same number of calories is not very effective for losing weight in the short term. There are two reasons that exercise alone doesn't work well. First, to lose even a small amount of weight just by exercising, you have to exercise a lot. Our bodies are very savvy about storing fat and conserving energy, and they function as if the next famine might start tomorrow. To burn 1 pound of fat, for example, you have to briskly walk or run 35 miles. Second, when most people exercise more, they unconsciously eat more. (There goes the body's self-preservation instinct again.) Result: a stalemate. If you exercise only, you'll be a lot fitter but not much lighter in the short term. The importance of exercise over the long term is a critically different story.

Combining calorie control and exercise. Here's the winner. Numerous studies have shown that combining a diet that restricts calories with regular exercise is the most effective way to lose weight for the short term. After active weight loss, following a balanced nutrition plan while continuing to exercise regularly is the most effective way to maintain the loss long-term. In one study, for example, which involved people who had lost at least 30 pounds and kept it off for at least 5 years, more than 90 percent had used the strategy of paying attention to their calorie intake while participating in regular physical activity.

This solution is not as intriguing, appealing, or sexy as the latest Metabo-Hypo-Glyco-Enzyme-Crunching 10-Day Miracle Weight-Loss Plan. But it has the scientific facts and the track record on its side.

CAN MEDICATIONS HELP?

Many medications to assist in weight loss have been tested in research laboratories, including mine, and there are others in the development pipeline. Within the next 10 years, we are going to see a whole host of medicines that will help people achieve long-term and safe weight loss. For those who have a lot of weight to lose, some of the medications currently available may be effective adjuncts to the lifestyle measures I've already discussed. You should, of course, consult your physician about the appropriateness of using such medication.

GETTING STARTED

Anyone who has tried to lose weight knows that it is not a trivial task. Over the years, however, I have seen many people succeed not only in losing weight but also in keeping it off. Here are some of the principles that my patients adopted that have allowed them to achieve long-term success.

Principle 1: You must burn more calories than you take in. As I've already stated, this is the bottom line. The medical literature is very clear that the combination of increasing physical activity and restricting calories is effective for both short-term weight loss and long-term maintenance.

Principle 2: It is virtually impossible to achieve permanent weight loss without consistent exercise. You know from previous chapters that I am a strong advocate of exercise, both for joint health and for overall health. When it comes to weight loss, it is very difficult to keep weight off if you do not make a fundamental decision to become more physically active. If you make that decision, you will also gain the many benefits of strengthening your joints and improving their general health.

Principle 3: View any weight loss that you maintain as a success. Remember that losing just 10 to 15 pounds, or 5 to 10 percent of your body weight, offers major health benefits for your joints, your heart, and the rest of your body. Some studies show that many people who try to lose weight are disappointed with what they view as "small" losses. Don't be. Celebrate your success. Maintain that new weight. Then later, when you are ready, work on losing and then maintaining another "small" loss for big benefits.

Principle 4: Adopt a lifelong strategy for a lifelong problem. You need to get away from short-term thinking. Most people who are overweight have battled weight throughout their lives. For lifelong maintenance of weight loss, it's important to find things that you can do on a daily basis to help you be aware of the amount of food—and often, the kinds of food—that you consume, as well as to increase physical activity. Anyone who has tried to lose weight knows that the key is not whether you can lose weight in the short term but whether you can keep it off. Adopt a long-term mindset.

THE RIGHT PLAN FOR YOU

Each year, a new book offering a "miracle" weight-loss system reaches the top of the best-seller list. Over the years, I have seen them all: the high-protein diet, the high-fat diet, the low-carbohydrate diet, the cabbage and grapefruit diets—you name it. In any given year, people will swear that that year's diet is the best ever devised. Then, the following year, something new comes along. The reason that there is something new each year is that none of these fad diets work long-term.

The best plan is one that focuses on an overall healthful diet and involves paying lifelong attention to portion control, eating real food with balanced nutrition, and getting regular physical activity. I recommend that you seek advice from a registered dietitian or join one of the reputable organizations, such as Weight Watchers, that can provide not only good information but also group support to help you lose weight. The walking and other physical activity and the stretching and strength-training programs of the 8-Week Joint Health Program can also help you reach your weight-loss goals.

Anyone who has tried to lose weight knows what a difficult challenge it is. If you are overweight, however, I urge you to make the effort. It can be one of the very best things that you do, not only to keep your joints healthy for life but also to improve your overall health and well-being.

Eating for Joint Health

Ever since I began my medical career, I have been involved in research as well as clinical practice. One of the most exciting aspects of research is the march of discovery. I mention this because there is a lot of ongoing research into the relationship of nutrition and diet to various aspects of health, including joint health. The issues and mechanisms being explored are very complex, but each year we learn more. In the past 10 years, in fact, solid scientific evidence has begun to emerge that various aspects of sound nutrition can have a significant impact on keeping your joints healthy or helping to decrease symptoms or improve function if you have joint problems, including osteoarthritis. (Evidence for these links may be even stronger for various inflammatory forms of arthritis, which we are only touching on in this book.) As a physician who keeps an open mind but insists on good scientific evidence (not just anecdotal experience), I could not have made that statement 10 years ago.

Of course, when it comes to food, we all eat—and feel strongly about what we eat. It seems to be common sense, based on what we know of how either good or poor nutrition influences both general health and particular aspects such as heart health, that nutrition would also have links to joint health and osteoarthritis. The soundness of the commonsense position, however, also opens the door to those who take advantage of health needs and the openness of the nutritional marketplace to promote "miracle cures" that have little or no scientific merit. In this briar patch, using your common sense and insisting on knowing the science can help you separate the helpful and promising information from the hype.

With that said, I am going to explore some of the possible links between nutrition and joint health in this chapter and the next on supplementation. I will also alert you to a few questionable or ineffective practices that have received publicity in the popular press, on various Web sites, and in chat rooms.

THE LINKS BETWEEN DIET AND JOINT HEALTH

If you want to establish a good foundation for joint health, the best place to start is with the nutritional practices recommended for overall health. Plan your meals using the following guidelines. These basic principles were developed on the basis of thousands of studies and have been recommended by the American Dietetic Association, American Diabetes Association, and American Heart Association, among other scientific groups. They are also consistent with the new nutritional guidelines for Americans issued by the USDA (on the Web at www.usda.gov/cnpp).

Moderate your fat intake. Consuming lots of fat, particularly saturated fat, is strongly linked to heart disease, high cholesterol, obesity, some cancers, and—here's the important point for joints—the body's inflammation response. Although inflammation is a greater problem in inflammatory arthritis such as rheumatoid arthritis than it is in osteoarthritis, limiting fat intake to the recommended level may be helpful for your joints, and it is certainly good health advice. The goal is to consume no more than 30 percent of your total calories from fat and no more than 10 percent from saturated fat, which is found primarily in animal products. Ounce for ounce, fat also has twice the calories of carbohydrates and proteins. Emphasize monounsaturated fats, which provide health benefits.

Lower your cholesterol consumption. By eating fewer cholesterol-rich foods and less saturated fat, you'll lower the amount of cholesterol in your blood, which contributes to heart disease. More important to the joints, cholesterol comes only from animal products, which may be generally high in fat (see above).

Eat more complex carbohydrates, particularly fruits, vegetables, and whole grains. These foods are high in vitamins, minerals, antioxidants, and phytochemicals that appear not only to contribute to health but also to actively fight the negative effects of free radicals. (Free radicals are unstable oxygen molecules in the body that damage cells and contribute to many of the conditions that are commonly linked with aging.) They are also the best sources of soluble and insoluble fiber. Make complex carbohydrates the base of your healthy eating plan, and eat sugar and sugary foods only in moderation.

Limit protein. Most Americans consume too much protein (particularly given the popularity of a certain fad diet). Our bodies need only about 15 percent of calories from protein. People who consume large amounts of protein usually get it from meats or other animal products that have fat and other components associated with the body's inflammatory response and weight gain. Many of these products are also rich in purine, the substance that can trigger attacks for people who suffer from gout, which is one kind of inflammatory arthritis.

Cut back on salt (sodium). Limiting your sodium intake to 2.4 grams (about 1 teaspoon of salt) a day can contribute to maintaining healthy blood pressure. Salt is found mainly in processed and prepared foods. Choose foods sensibly and use herbs, spices, and fruit instead of salt to boost flavor.

If you consume alcohol, do so in moderation. Moderate alcohol consumption is defined as no more than one drink per day for women and no more than two drinks per day for men (one drink is equal to 1.5 ounces of distilled spirits, one 5-ounce glass of wine, or 12 ounces of beer). Drinking more than this may raise the risk of heart attack and is associated with weight gain, high blood pressure, liver disease, and gout.

Do not consume more calories than required to maintain a healthy body weight. As I have noted frequently, excess weight places major destructive stress on your joints, not to mention the increased risk it poses for heart disease, high blood pressure, diabetes, stroke, and certain cancers. Following the previous steps can do a lot to help you meet this guideline.

Consume a variety of foods. A balanced intake of all types of foods ensures that you get a wide range of nutrients, including the essential vitamins and minerals as well as antioxidants, flavonoids, and phytochemicals. Consult the Nutrition Facts labels on foods to identify healthful choices. Eliminating any category of food (carbohydrate, protein, or fat) permanently is not a good approach. It's not hard for most people to accommodate any food sensitivities and still get a balanced diet. The obstacles are that discomfort from joint pain may make you less likely to prepare balanced meals and that some medications for joint pain and problems may depress your appetite. So work with your physician and a nutrition professional to overcome these roadblocks on the way to healthful eating.

Drink plenty of water. Some of the official nutrition guidelines allude to this important practice but don't mention it directly, so think of it as Rippe's Rule. Maintaining proper hydration is one of the most neglected health principles, and lots of people live life in a state of mild dehydration. Yet the human body is largely composed of water, and we lose up to a gallon a day. Being dehydrated by lack of as little as a quart of water makes you feel and perform less than your best both mentally and physically. Drinking plenty of water also helps your body eliminate substances that may contribute to inflammation.

Proper hydration is particularly important as you carry out the activity programs of the 8-Week Joint Health Program, so drink before, during, and after activity. If you wait until you feel thirsty, it's too late.

NUTRITIONAL PRACTICES TO PROMOTE JOINT HEALTH

Among the various areas that are under investigation, I believe that there are three in which the evidence suggests that some practices may lessen the impact of joint disease as well as promote good joint health.

A PROPER MIXTURE OF OILS

As already mentioned, certain fats may contribute to the inflammatory component of arthritis. The saturated fats found in a variety of animal products and particularly in red meat, for example, may contribute to the inflammatory process. In addition to saturated fat, however, the omega-6 fatty acids, which are common in vegetable oils such as corn and safflower oils and are also used in many processed and fast foods, have also been shown to potentially contribute to joint inflammation. This is of particular concern to people who have rheumatoid arthritis and other forms of inflammatory arthritis.

My recommendation is to substitute monounsaturated fats for saturated fats when possible. Also, when possible, you should substitute

Fat Sources

Monounsaturated fats can be found in the following foods.

- Olives and olive oil
- Canola oil
- Avocados and avocado oil
- Peanuts, peanut butter, and peanut oil
- Pecans

Here's where to find omega-3 fatty acids.

- Sardines*
- Flaxseed oil*
- Mackerel*
- Herring*
- Lake trout
- Sablefish*
- Salmon* (wild, not farmed)
- Bluefish
- Mullet

These are common sources of omega-6 fatty acids.

- Corn oil
- Safflower oil
- Sunflower oil
- Most processed snack foods
- Meat from corn-fed animals

*These foods are high in total fat and thus in total calories.

omega-3 fatty acids for omega-6 fatty acids. How do you do this? Olive oil is an excellent, great-tasting source of monounsaturated fat, and cold-water fish supplies omega-3's. See "Fat Sources" for more information.

A VEGETARIAN DIET

Many more people are now contemplating vegetarian diets. Some follow a strict vegetarian diet, called a vegan diet, that includes no animal products. Others follow a modified vegetarian diet that includes some animal products, such as eggs or dairy products and sometimes fish.

The principles of a vegetarian diet may work to improve joint health. At the very least, they are likely to increase your intake of antioxidants and vitamins because you consume more fruits and vegetables. Unfortunately, the average American consumes far fewer than the recommended minimum of five fruits and vegetables daily. If you are thinking of adopting a vegetarian diet to promote joint health, I would strongly recommend that you speak to a registered dietitian. Later in this chapter, you will learn the best sources of nutritional advice.

LOW-PURINE DIET FOR GOUT

Gout, a form of arthritis that causes joint inflammation, is the one form of joint disease for which a nutritional component has been clearly proven. For centuries, gout was considered an affliction of the well-to-do because they were the only people who could afford to eat a rich diet that included meat, wine, and beer, among other foods. Now we know that people who have gout have either a problem eliminating uric acid or a defect that causes the body to make too much uric acid. Some of the building blocks of uric acid, called purines, come from foods such as meat and some fish. Today, we have excellent medicines to treat gout, but if you are subject to problems with gouty arthritis, it is very wise to follow a nutritional plan that is low in meats (particularly organ meats) and also in certain types of seafood, such as anchovies, sardines, and mackerel. You should also avoid excessive alcohol consumption and drink plenty of water.

VITAMINS AND JOINT HEALTH

In the past decade, a great deal of evidence has accumulated that certain types of vitamins, which we call antioxidants, can contribute to both general good health and joint health. The vitamins that fall into this class are beta-carotene (a precursor of vitamin A), vitamin C, and vitamin E. Vitamin D is also important because it helps regulate the growth, hardening, and repair of bones by contributing to the absorption of calcium. And vitamin K helps by activating at least three proteins that are needed for bone health.

We know that one of the components of arthritis is inflammation of the joint. We now believe that free radicals can contribute to joint inflammation. For this reason, it makes a great deal of sense to be sure that you eat a diet rich in the fruits and vegetables that contain antioxidants. In addition, it makes sense to supplement with these vitamins in cases where your intake may be low.

Vitamin C. Vitamin C helps in the production of collagen, a necessary component of cartilage and connective tissues. In the Framingham Osteoarthritis Study, people who got additional vitamin C, either from supplements or in diets that had considerable amounts of citrus fruits or other foods high in vitamin C (such as certain green vegetables), had a significantly decreased risk of developing joint inflammation and arthritis.

The beneficial results, it is thought, may be due to both vitamin C's antioxidant function and the role it plays in the production of collagen and thus in joint health. The product tested in our joint health study included vitamin C. Participants who consumed the recommended serving of 10 grams of the gelatin-based supplement received 60 milligrams of vitamin C, which is the Daily Value (DV). Consuming this amount of vitamin C (the amount in one orange or ¾ cup of grapefruit juice) is a good nutritional practice to promote joint health. Besides citrus fruits and juices, kiwifruit, broccoli, brussels sprouts, and red bell peppers provide significant amounts.

Beta-carotene, vitamin A, and vitamin D. In addition to the ability of beta-carotene to fight the oxidative damage of free radicals, vitamins A and D play roles in the development of strong bones. Just how and how much these vitamins may contribute to joint health is under investigation. Meanwhile, remember that in larger doses, vitamin A is toxic, so I would not recommend that you consume more than the DV (5,000 IU). You can get good amounts of beta-carotene by eating brightly colored fruits and vegetables such as spinach, carrots, cantaloupe, and apricots; preformed vitamin A is available from animal products such as beef liver and milk. For vitamin D, look for fortified milk and cereals. The DV is 400 IU.

Vitamin E. Vitamin E is a very strong antioxidant that appears to protect cellular membranes and cell components from oxidative damage. It's difficult to get the DV (30 IU) from foods, so your physician may recommend that you take vitamin E as a supplement for several reasons, including joint health.

Ongoing research. Research is just beginning to unveil the complex roles that these and other vitamins and minerals play in joint health and other aspects of health. For now, I would recommend that you eat a diet that is rich in all these nutrients, which means a diet rich in fruits, vegetables, and whole grains. If you do not get the DVs for these nutrients from your diet, it's probably a good idea to supplement to those levels. Before supplementing in higher amounts, it would be wise to consult your physician or a registered dietitian.

POSSIBLE LINKS BETWEEN DIET AND JOINT DISEASE

There is a growing body of literature that suggests that there may actually be some relationship between dietary habits and joint disease, particularly the inflammatory forms of arthritis. A small number of people who have arthritis or other joint problems, for example, may be sensitive to certain foods that can trigger symptoms such as inflammation or make them worse. As noted earlier, it is also possible that a diet high in certain foods, such as saturated animal fats, may affect the inflammatory response, which in turn may contribute to worsening the inflammatory component of arthritis.

From a practical perspective, there is no question that joint problems can make your diet worse. People who suffer from significant arthritis may have difficulty shopping and preparing food, and, in extreme cases, they may also have difficulty chewing and eating. Furthermore, constant pain and the fatigue that may accompany it can wreck your appetite. These potential problems offer more good reasons to take steps to enhance joint health and function as soon as you can.

BE WARY OF QUESTIONABLE DIETARY PLANS

If you already have joint problems, you know that many people tout various nutritional practices to help with arthritis or other joint problems. Here are some to be cautious about.

Fad diets. If you hear of a new "arthritis diet," be careful if it stresses only one food or a few foods and suggests that you totally eliminate other types or groups of foods. Be skeptical also if the effectiveness of a diet is demonstrated by testimonials (even if the person doing the "testifying" is a physician or scientist), rather than being based on reputable scientific evidence, or if the scientific evidence or support seems inadequate. Be particularly wary of diets that claim to "cure" arthritis, because the only known types of arthritis that can be cured are gout, bacterial arthritis, and Lyme disease. Finally, beware of hype. There are some diets out there that are built on promising ideas, but the claims have been inflated beyond what the evidence to date will support. Use your common sense to separate the promising from the proven.

Fasting. Fasting has been advocated by some to relieve or cure arthritis. While some studies show that some people with rheumatoid arthritis may experience temporary relief with limited fasts of a day or so, after the fast, the symptoms return and may even worsen. There is no evidence that fasting helps osteoarthritis or other joint problems. I do not recommend fasting for joint health. Repeated or prolonged fasting can actually cause a significant increase in problems from joint disease and may also lead to malnutrition, which is bad for your joints and overall health. If limited, occasional fasting (in which you consume water and juice but no solid food) is part of your religious or spiritual tradition, however, there should be no problem.

Dairy-free diets. A small percentage of people, whether they have joint problems or not, lack an enzyme called lactase that is needed to digest the sugar (lactose) in dairy products. This condition is called lactose intolerance. These people need to either take supplements to replace the missing enzyme or be very careful about consuming dairy products. Although a few studies have shown that some people with rheumatoid arthritis show improvement after removing dairy products from their diets, there is no evidence that doing this has any benefit at all for osteoarthritis. Furthermore, if you eliminate dairy products, you eliminate a major source of calcium and possibly contribute to bone problems. If you think that you may be sensitive to dairy products, try eliminating them from your diet for 1 week. Most people will notice no change in their joint symptoms.

Nightshade-free diet. Certain vegetables, such as tomatoes, peppers, and potatoes, are in the nightshade family, also known by the botanical name of Solanaceae. While diets that eliminate such foods have been recommended for people with certain kinds of arthritis, particularly rheumatoid arthritis, there is no clear scientific evidence to support this practice.

IS THERE AN ARTHRITIS DIET?

Although many dietary practices may enhance joint comfort and health for various people with various types of joint disease, there is no one "arthritis diet." Popular books may use the title to promote everything from a generally sound eating plan to diets that can be downright dangerous to health. I am particularly concerned about diets that eliminate whole categories of foods. Under the guidance of a physician who's trying to identify a patient's food sensitivities and allergies, supervised elimination diets have a valid role, and, I might add, can take months to complete. The so-called elimination diets promoted by popular books and media often have not a shred of scientific evidence behind them. I would avoid these entirely.

FINDING EXPERT RESOURCES

If you are contemplating improving your nutrition, the best place to start is with some expert advice. Every patient I see is also seen by a registered dietitian. I highly recommend this practice. Registered dietitians go through a rigorous training process that helps them understand and recommend real foods for real people. Usually, a dietitian charges $50 to $75 an hour for a consultation. It is money well spent.

The best source of information about registered dietitians is the American Dietetic Association (ADA), which can also provide links to other objective sources. The explosion of information available on the Internet as well as in the print media presents a real challenge in determining which information is objective and which promotes a particular product or point of view. So get some help. You can reach the ADA by calling (800) 366-1655 for recorded messages. The association also has a good Web site at www.eatright.org.

For sorting through the substantial amount of information on nutrition that's available on the Internet, another good place to start is with a search engine called Nutrition Navigator, which is produced and run by the nutrition department at Tufts University in Boston. You can check www.navigator.tufts.edu/ for regular updates and objective ratings of other nutrition sites on the Web.

Nutrition and good health are linked. After all, as the *Surgeon General's Report on Nutrition* told us, 8 out of the 10 leading causes of death in the United States have a nutrition or alcohol component. If your goal is to improve your joint health or your general health, starting with nutrition is a very good idea. This is an area where "knowledge is power," so try to become as knowledgeable as possible on what works and what does not. You can make an enormous difference in your joint health and your overall health by following the general nutritional principles outlined here and obtained from other reputable sources.

Using Supplements Wisely

Throughout *The Joint Health Prescription*, I have been talking about simple things that each of us can do to maintain healthy joints throughout a lifetime or to reduce the symptoms of existing joint problems. The important core recommendations include performing regular physical activity, engaging in a regular program of stretching, strengthening your muscles, taking appropriate precautions to avoid traumatic injuries to the joints, maintaining a proper body weight, and eating a nutritionally balanced diet. All of these practices make up your primary program for joint health and a main defense against joint pain.

Over the past decade, growing scientific evidence has suggested that certain nutritional supplements may also play a role in helping to maintain joint health and alleviate joint pain. Here, I will discuss the most prominent of these products, including gelatin-based supplements, glucosamine, chondroitin, and others, and review the evidence—pro, con, or not yet proved—for the claims of their benefits. The positive effects on joint health of the antioxidant vitamins—vitamins C and E and beta-carotene—are discussed in chapter 9.

CAVEAT EMPTOR

This Latin phrase—"let the buyer beware"—says it all when it comes to supplementation and health, for both general health and joint health. There are some wonderful supplements on the market, including some that I feel comfortable in recommending as adjuncts for maintaining and enhancing joint health. However, the field of nutritional supplements has little regulation and few quality-control safeguards.

Nutritional supplements are regulated under a 1994 federal law called the Dietary Supplement Health Education Act (DSHEA). Its purpose was to encourage ethical companies to investigate the potential health benefits of natural products that were already part of the normal food chain and were generally regarded as safe. Many reputable companies began to explore these products and to develop supplements based on previous significant scientific studies. But the act also opened the door to fast-buck companies that simply marketed a product and touted its benefits without any scientific background and often without adequate quality control.

How did they get away with this? Easily. Under the DSHEA, products sold as dietary supplements don't have to meet the same standards of safety and efficacy that are required of pharmaceutical agents, which are regulated by the FDA. Although the companies that sell the supplements are not supposed to claim that they can cure or treat any problem or disease (only that they support health), ambiguous wording on the packaging often implies otherwise. Some retailers who sell the products are often even more direct. Whether you think that such an open marketplace is positive or negative, this freedom means that the buyer must truly beware.

One of the best ways to ensure quality is to find out as much as you can about the supplement company. Check how long it's been in business, whether it has a reputable medical advisory board, whether it underwrites or conducts research, and if it distributes quality educational materials. Here are some other factors to consider.

■ Be aware that the product may be contaminated and/or may not contain exactly the ingredients or strengths listed on the label. Independent testing has often shown that supplements, particularly herbals, contain impurities or plant products besides those listed as ingredients. Because of the way plants grow and are harvested, it is not easy to ensure that other substances don't get mixed in. The active ingredients may also be of higher or lower strengths than what is listed on the label. Don't purchase a product whose label does not list all ingredients and their potency. Again, your best strategy is to buy products from reputable companies that test and stand behind their products.

- Remember that you can't tell the quality of a product by its package. These days, all products, whatever the form (capsules, tablets, tea bags, powders, and so on), come in sophisticated packaging. Packaging has nothing to do with quality.
- Consider possible negative interactions with medicines or other supplements that you may be taking. Just because a product is "natural" does not mean that it is not a powerful drug or that it's safe to take with anything else. About 25 percent of our modern drugs, including powerful narcotics, for example, come from plants. Be sure to tell your physician what supplements you are taking and ask about possible interactions. Also, if you're interested in trying a new supplement, your doctor may be able to recommend a brand.

On the positive side, more companies are beginning to make sure that their products undergo independent scientific testing by laboratories such as mine. Here are some of the available supplements and the evidence that may link them to improved joint health.

GELATIN-BASED SUPPLEMENTS

Gelatin-based supplements—most of which are designed to be added to beverages—are among the most promising nutritional supports for joint health. As I mentioned in chapter 2, the results for people in our study who took this type of supplement were very impressive. Although all participants (including the control group) showed decreased joint pain and improved mobility and quality of life, participants who took the gelatin-based supplement had significant improvement in knee function—measured with high-tech methods—compared to those who took placebos.

What are the active ingredients? The supplement used in the study is a combination of gelatin, vitamin C, and calcium. Gelatin, also known by its scientific name, hydrolyzed collagen protein (HCP), is naturally occurring but not vegetarian. The supplement is formulated to dissolve in beverages without congealing as regular cooking gelatin does. The daily serving, usually taken in the morning for convenience, is 10 grams of hydrolyzed gelatin mixed in a noncarbonated, nonalcoholic drink of your choice. In our test, the positive results started to become apparent by 8 weeks and were clearly apparent by 14 weeks.

How do the supplements work? Cartilage in the joints has high concentrations of two amino acids, glycine and proline. Because blood supply to the cartilage is poor, however, these basic building blocks for maintaining the cartilage in good health or repairing it when it is injured may be in short supply. Because gelatin contains high levels of glycine and proline, the theory is that the product increases the availability of these amino acids and helps the cartilage to remain healthy.

Vitamin C was included in the formula that we tested because data from the Framingham Osteoarthritis Study and others suggest that the antioxidant properties of vitamin C help reduce joint inflammation. People in the Framingham study who had an increased intake of vitamin C had a decreased incidence of osteoarthritis. The 60 milligrams of vitamin C included in a serving of the supplement used in our study is 100 percent of the Daily Value (DV) for vitamin C.

Calcium was included in the formula because it helps maintain the structural integrity and therefore the strength of bones. The 150 milligrams included in a serving of the supplement we tested is 15 percent of the DV.

Gelatin-based supplements appear to have very few side effects, none of which are significant or worrisome. In our study, 95 percent of the participants who took either the supplements or the placebos had no side effects. Among the remaining 5 percent, minor symptoms were reported, such as a feeling of fullness or bloating. There was no significant difference between groups in the reports of symptoms.

My overall conclusion is that this is a product that really works. For this reason, I recommend taking a gelatin-based supplement with 10 grams of hydrolyzed gelatin as one of the mainstays of a program to maintain good joint health.

GLUCOSAMINE

Glucosamine has been touted as a "cure" for arthritis. Although this is certainly an overstatement, studies show that glucosamine does help to ease the pain and stiffness of osteoarthritis. Research is ongoing to determine whether it can actually maintain or promote joint health.

Glucosamine is a form of sugar that is a basic building block of several chemicals that are important components of the cartilage in joints. It is a natural substance that is extracted from crab, lobster, or shrimp shells. Early in 2001, the medical journal *Lancet* reported on a 3-year study conducted in Belgium with people who had mild to moderate osteoarthritis in their knees. The study showed that glucosamine decreased the subjects' symptoms and prevented further joint damage. In addition, a large, rigidly controlled test conducted by the National Institutes of Health is currently investigating glucosamine's role in improving osteoarthritis symptoms.

The usual dose of glucosamine is 1,500 milligrams a day. Testing to date shows that it takes about 2 months to notice benefits. There are few side effects, but people with diabetes or shellfish allergies should consult their doctors before trying it.

A few gelatin-based supplements have added glucosamine. Glucosamine is also often combined with chondroitin (see below). The good news is that it, too, has very few side effects, so it appears reasonable to take as a supplement if you already have symptoms of osteoarthritis.

CHONDROITIN

Chondroitin exists naturally in cartilage in the joints and is thought to make your cartilage more supple and to protect it from destructive enzymes. It has been used in both animals and humans to relieve symptoms of osteoarthritis for many years. The recommended dose is 1,200 milligrams a day. Although chondroitin is most often taken in combination with glucosamine, there are no studies that show that the combination is any more effective than either of them taken alone. Chondroitin has minimal side effects and may be worth a try, but some people don't respond to it at all. If you have used it for 2 to 3 months and have gotten no response, it probably is not worth continuing.

CAT'S CLAW

Cat's claw (*Uncaria tomentosa*) is a vine that grows in the wilds of the Peruvian jungle, along the Amazon River. It's important to know its botanical name because there are other cat's claw plants that are toxic. The herb has a long tradition in Peruvian folk medicine as a treatment for inflammation and bone pain and is traditionally taken in the form of tea made by boiling the bark of the vine. A typical dose is 500 to 1,000 milligrams three times a day. It is sold in tea bags and in capsules. At this point, even though it is widely used in South America, there are no human studies to show that it works. People who are taking blood-thinning drugs (anticoagulants) should also be very cautious, since cat's claw can increase the risk of bleeding.

DHEA

DHEA (short for dehydroepiandrosterone) is a mild male hormone that is produced naturally by the body and forms the basis for a number of sex hormones, including testosterone and estrogen. DHEA has been touted as a cure for a wide variety of conditions ranging from cancer to aging. Its only possible use for joint pain is for lupus, a type of inflammatory arthritis, and this application is currently being studied.

The sources of DHEA vary widely in potency. Because it is a hormone, DHEA can create tremendous problems in the body. I would not recommend that you take it for any reason without discussing it in detail with your physician.

DMSO

DMSO, or dimethyl sulfoxide, is a by-product of wood processing that is used primarily as an industrial solvent and an ingredient in antifreeze. It also has legitimate medical uses in veterinary medicine and some human applications. Applied externally, this chemical has the ability to transport itself and anything it contacts across cell membranes, through the skin, and into internal tissues. Anyone who has ever played an active sport has probably at least heard of this drug, which has been touted for its ability to relieve the aches and strains of sport and to leave your breath tasting and smelling as if you'd eaten a chemical factory.

DMSO is a very powerful substance, and I cannot recommend using it without medical supervision. If you are thinking about trying it to treat your arthritis, you should consult your physician first. Self-treatment, particularly if you don't acquire the medically pure product, can be dangerous.

FISH OIL

Fish oil, particularly oils from cold-water fish such as mackerel and salmon, may help relieve arthritis symptoms by reducing inflammation and pain. Fish oil is high in omega-3 fatty acids and has also been shown to lower the risk of heart attack. The usual dose is 3 grams (3,000 milligrams) of omega-3's.

Although fish oil may be beneficial for joint health, be careful, because the number of capsules that you need to take (10 to 15 a day) may contain a lot of calories, and you could easily see your weight start creeping up. Most of the benefits of fish oil can also be obtained by eating fish. If you take blood-thinning drugs, be sure to consult your physician before taking fish oil, because it also is a blood thinner and could produce complications.

FLAXSEED

Flaxseed is somewhat similar to fish oil in the sense that it contains a type of omega-3 oil called EPA that is thought to be good for arthritis. Studies that might prove this have not yet been conducted, however. A typical recommendation for people who wish to take flaxseed to improve symptoms of osteoarthritis is 1 to 3 tablespoons a day of the oil or 30 grams (¼ cup) of flax meal. I don't believe that there is enough evidence at this point, though, to strongly recommend flaxseed, even to reduce the symptoms of osteoarthritis.

HERBAL COX-2 INHIBITORS

Celecoxib (Celebrex) and rofecoxib (Vioxx) may be the best-known members of a relatively new class of pharmaceuticals called COX-2 inhibitors. They're said to relieve pain as effectively as traditional nonsteroidal anti-inflammatory drugs (NSAIDs), but they're less likely to cause the gastrointestinal distress and other side effects associated with their predecessors.

Some herbs contain compounds that may work somewhat like the pharmaceutical COX-2's. For example, curcumin—the yellow pigment in turmeric—has potent anti-inflammatory and pain-relieving properties. To treat osteoarthritis, some experts recommend taking 400 milligrams three times a day. Follow the dosage directions on the product that you choose.

Other herbs that have these compounds include feverfew, ginger, green tea, rosemary, skullcap, and thyme.

MSM

Methylsulfonylmethane, popularly known as MSM, has gotten a lot of attention as an arthritis treatment. To date, the evidence supporting its pain-relieving properties comes only from anecdotal reports.

In theory, MSM reduces the inflammation of arthritis by increasing the effectiveness of cortisol, the body's own anti-inflammatory compound. MSM is a component of dimethyl sulfoxide (DMSO) but produces far fewer side effects.

Only a few scientific studies have attempted to assess MSM's pain-relieving potential, and none of them have been published. That said, the supplement appears safe, even in doses as large as 8,000 milligrams a day.

Some experts recommend starting with 1,000 milligrams a day, though your best bet is to follow the dosage guidelines on the label of the product you choose. MSM does have a mild blood-thinning effect, so it should not be used with pharmaceutical blood thinners, including aspirin. It also takes time to work—at least 4 weeks, if not longer.

SAM-E

Perhaps best-known as an antidepressant, SAM-e (S-adenosyl-L-methionine) has also shown promise as an osteoarthritis treatment. Specifically, it stimulates the production of chondrocytes and proteoglycans, which help rebuild worn or damaged cartilage in joints. In one study involving 20,000 people with arthritis, about 80 percent of those who took SAM-e reported significant pain relief. The recommended dosage is 600 to 1,200 milligrams a day, taken in three doses of 200 to 400 milligrams each.

SHARK CARTILAGE

The argument for taking cartilage of any kind (from sharks, chickens, or other sources) in capsules or pills to ease the symptoms of osteoarthritis may seem logical. If your cartilage is damaged, why not take supplements of cartilage to help fix it? At this time, however, there is insufficient evidence that shark cartilage is safe and effective for treating joint problems.

There is some mixed and controversial evidence that shark cartilage, unlike other types, may be useful in treating cancer tumors because it suppresses the creation of new blood vessels and thus blood flow to the tumor. Until more is known about this potential for blood vessel suppression, I would not use shark cartilage at all for self-care.

DISCUSSING SUPPLEMENTS WITH YOUR DOCTOR

When I see patients at my clinic, I always ask them if they are taking vitamins, minerals, or other supplements. More than half of the adult population in the United States is currently taking at least one supplement, yet less than 25 percent of them have ever discussed it with their doctors. This is a mistake. If you are taking supplements, whether for joint health or any other reason, it is important to let your doctor know, because many supplements may either interact with prescription medicines that you are taking or have side effects of their own.

THE ROLE OF SUPPLEMENTS IN JOINT HEALTH

In the past 5 years, and particularly now that my research institute has completed its study, a role for supplementation has been steadily emerging. I believe that we can now safely say that for many people, particularly those who have mild symptoms of joint discomfort, taking gelatin-based supplements can enhance joint health. Glucosamine or chondroitin may also be beneficial, particularly for people who have symptoms of osteoarthritis. When it comes to the rest of the supplements, the data is incomplete in many instances, and in some cases, there is very little data at all to support taking them for joint health. I am always on the lookout for naturally occurring substances that can provide health benefits, but this is an area where I would urge you to be cautious and look for clear-cut scientific evidence, such as that provided by our study. It is also very important when you are investigating supplements to look for manufacturers with good reputations for quality control.

Maintaining Healthy Joints for Life

f you have reached this chapter, you have at least read all about, if not started, the 8-Week Joint Health Program. As you can see, the program offers you a "laboratory" where you can begin to practice, experiment with, and customize for your personal needs all the daily habits and activities that you can use throughout your life to promote joint health. Practices such as regular physical activity, strength training, flexibility exercises, good nutrition, and, in many instances, supplementation can make a huge difference in the health of your joints.

By starting the 8-Week Joint Health Program, you have implemented what I call a lifestyle approach to joint health. Together, the program and the principles of lifestyle medicine provide a 10-step, lifetime strategy for maintaining healthy joints. The steps that follow not only provide excellent preventive medicine for your joints, they also can help you decrease the pain and other symptoms of existing joint disease, such as osteoarthritis, and improve your functioning and quality of life.

STEP 1: MAKE A COMMITMENT

If you make a commitment before you have serious joint problems and then follow through with a specific plan such as that outlined in this book, you can do a lot to keep your joints healthy for years to come. If you already have mild joint problems or perhaps an old injury that makes later problems more likely, making a commitment now is even more important.

STEP 2: ESTABLISH A REGULAR WALKING PROGRAM

Following a regular walking program is one of the very best ways to prevent or ease joint pain and stiffness and to maintain and promote joint health. Walking is low-impact, flexible, and simple, and it requires little equipment. It nourishes the cartilage, synovial fluid, and other structures of the joints, particularly in the lower body, and strengthens the muscles that help cushion and support the joints.

Of course, other forms of aerobic exercise are also beneficial, but as a practical matter, walking remains my number one recommendation. It would keep everyone healthier overall while also promoting excellent joint health. So, if you want to use another form of aerobic activity such as jogging, cycling, or swimming, that's fine, but don't ignore walking. (See chapter 5.)

STEP 3: INCREASE DAILY PHYSICAL ACTIVITY

Walking, although wonderful, is only one of many forms of physical activity. An active lifestyle is a healthy lifestyle; *inactivity* is hazardous to your health. The key message is not to try to turn your life upside down; that's a recipe for burning out and collapsing into the same old rut. Rather, look for nooks and crannies here and there in your life where you can add a few minutes of physical activity. Make a commitment to planting a garden this year, for instance. It will be good not only for your joints but also for your mental outlook, and it will give you a sense of accomplishment. Park farther away from the stores when you shop. Take the stairs at work. Get up and dance or do a few toe raises during television commercials. Think "movement." Think "activity." (See chapter 6.)

STEP 4: ESTABLISH A REGULAR STRETCHING PROGRAM

Stretching is wonderful for the joints. It takes the joints through a full range of motion and enables each joint to be limber enough to perform the activities that it was meant to perform. One problem that people experience as they reach their forties, fifties, and beyond is that their muscles become weak and their joints stiff because they are not physically active and don't stretch. This means that even a small extra exertion such as picking up your grandchild or playing tennis on the weekend can cause a major joint injury. So keep those joints limber and flexible with a regular stretching program. (See chapter 7.)

STEP 5: ESTABLISH A REGULAR STRENGTH-TRAINING PROGRAM

Many people don't realize the complex interaction between muscles and joints. Muscles help keep joints in position and help cushion impact. Because strong muscles are vital to healthy joints, I advocate a regular, total-body strength-training program. Even if you already have joint problems, a personal trainer or a physical therapist can modify strength-training programs to help you strengthen the muscles around injured or arthritic joints and restore function and comfort. (See chapter 7.)

STEP 6: MAINTAIN A HEALTHY BODY WEIGHT

Carrying too much weight can seriously stress and even injure the weight-bearing joints in our bodies. When you run, you land with three times your body weight on each stride, so think of all the excess pounding that your joints take if you gain weight. Being even 20 or 30 pounds overweight can result in thousands of pounds of extra pressure on a joint over the course of even 1 day.

Obesity is the leading cause of arthritis in women and the second leading cause (behind prior sports injuries) of arthritis in men in the United States. Make an effort to adopt practices such as healthy eating and regular physical activity that are vital to maintaining a healthy body weight. If you are overweight, speak to your physician, a registered dietitian, or an exercise physiologist about steps that you can take in your daily life to lose weight. (See chapter 8.) Maintaining a healthy weight is another of the best things you can do to keep your joints healthy and functioning as they should.

STEP 7: EAT A HEALTHFUL DIET

Don't underestimate the links between nutrition and joint health. Following the USDA's nutritional guidelines for Americans promotes joint health in addition to overall health. (See chapter 9.) Depending on the condition of your joints, you may need to make a few modifications, such as paying particular attention to the types of oils that you consume. Cut down on corn oil and other oils that contain a lot of linoleic acid and focus on oils such as fish oils, which contain omega-3 oils. Substituting monounsaturated fats, such as olive oil, for saturated fats is also good for both joint health and overall health. And, of course, one of the benefits of a healthy diet is that it helps you to maintain a healthy body weight.

STEP 8: CONSIDER SUPPLEMENTATION

Based on the findings of my study of joint health, taking supplements may be one of the important practices that you can adopt. Simply taking 10 grams of a high-quality hydrolyzed gelatin-based supplement in a beverage every day can make a difference in joint health. If you already have joint problems, other supplements such as glucosamine and chondroitin may also be helpful. (See chapter 10.)

STEP 9: AVOID INJURIES

Previous joint injuries are the leading cause of arthritis in men in the United States, and women have their share, too. I often see patients in my clinic who have bad knees or ankles because of traumatic injuries suffered in sports or other activities.

Maintaining a high overall fitness level is one of the most effective things you can do to minimize the likelihood of injury. People who are fit don't fatigue as quickly, and they have strong muscles, good flexibility, and good balance—all attributes that help prevent injuries.

If you play a sport, it's equally important to use proper technique. If you don't have the proper skills for a sport you're interested in, it would be a wise investment to have instruction in the correct biomechanical motion for that sport.

One other issue, which is covered in chapter 16, is which sports activity you choose. A great deal of medical literature suggests that some sports, particularly the so-called contact sports, are much more likely to cause joint injuries than noncontact sports. So if you do not have joint problems and are thinking about the kinds of activities that you may want to participate in, pick those with a low potential of injury. Of course, if you already have a joint injury, you should seek medical advice and participate in a proper program of rehabilitation to keep the problem from becoming chronic.

One final point is important to mention. There have been incredibly important advances in sports medicine techniques over the past decade. Many people don't realize that chronic joint injuries that in the past might have required major surgery can now be corrected with arthroscopic procedures. So if you have an injury and are looking for ways to get back in the game, consult your physician, who can refer you to an orthopedist with a special interest in sports medicine.

STEP 10: MAINTAIN YOUR STRATEGY FOR LIFE

Your joints are designed to give you a lifetime of mobility, so it is important to adopt a lifelong strategy to keep them healthy. The good news is that all of these steps—regular walking, proper nutrition, maintenance of proper body weight, and the others—will also promote general good health. If you carry out the 10 steps, you could decrease your risk of joint injury and maximize the healthy, pain-free function of your joints for life.

The Joint Owner's Maintenance Manual

Medical Evaluation of Your Joints

One of the key components of maintaining good joint health throughout your life is to establish a sound, working relationship with your physician. There are number of reasons why. First, a thorough check of not only your joints but also your musculoskeletal system can help identify trouble spots before they become real problems. Second, if a joint becomes painful, stiff, or otherwise troublesome, a good examination by a competent physician is an important first step toward getting proper treatment. Third, if you injure a joint, evaluation by a physician and sometimes a specialist such as a rheumatologist, orthopedist, or physical therapist can ensure that you get adequate treatment and rehabilitation to restore the joint to the best, most functional condition possible.

ROUTINE EXAMINATIONS

When you have your annual routine physical examination, you should take the opportunity to ask your physician for an evaluation of your musculoskeletal system and your joints. A regular checkup is one of the best ways to ensure that you keep your joints and muscles in tiptop shape. Here are some of the things that your physician will look for in a comprehensive joint and musculoskeletal examination.

In response to your request to evaluate your joints for potential problems such as arthritis, your doctor may ask if anything in particular is causing your concern. Maybe you're getting a little older and are concerned about osteoarthritis. Maybe your knee has been a little stiff in the morning or an old joint injury has recently caused twinges of pain. Maybe you've simply read this book and want to be sure to do all that you can to keep your joints healthy. By asking your reasons, your doctor has begun a very important part of the exam—the history, which has several parts.

Preventive history. First, your physician will review whether you have had any trauma to a joint or have any congenital abnormalities (structural differences in any joint or part of your musculoskeletal system that you were born with). It is very important to tell your doctor about when any joint trauma occurred or when or if you noticed a change in any congenital abnormality.

Symptomatic history. Your physician will then ask about your present problems with a specific joint or joints. Be sure to describe any pain or tenderness that you experience at rest or during activity. Your doctor will also ask you about other symptoms, such as the following.

- Recent swelling of a joint or the surrounding area
- Changes in skin color around a joint
- Joint stiffness in the morning or after the joint has been immobile for a period of time (a condition often called the gel phenomenon)
- Any grinding noises or sensations in your joints (called crepitus)
- Discomfort in the joint related to specific activities

Past medical history. Your physician will ask about your general past medical history, including your family medical history.

Social history. No, your physician does not need to know if you're a party animal but rather if your joint problem is affecting your work or domestic life or your ability to take care of yourself. And, sure, if the problem is keeping you from doing what you love, such as going out dancing or bowling every Friday night, share that fact, too.

Physical exam. After taking a thorough history, your doctor will do a general examination, including a check of your body temperature, blood pressure, and weight, and determine whether you have had recent exposure to diseases such as Lyme disease, which can cause arthritis. If you have a current joint problem, the doctor will continue with a physical examination of the joint.

EVALUATION OF ACUTE JOINT PROBLEMS

Whether a problem with a joint is discovered during a routine checkup or you go to your physician with an acute problem, such as an achy shoulder or a knee that's buckling, the doctor will take a history and then evaluate your symptoms and look for signs that will help diagnose the problem accurately. An evaluation of the area around the joint will determine whether your problem is related to the joint or to the bones or soft tissue in the area. This evaluation includes inspection and palpation.

Inspection. Your physician will compare the affected joint with its counterpart (for example, your right knee with your left knee), looking for differences in size, color, and bone structure.

Palpation. Next, your doctor will palpate (touch and manipulate) the joint to identify the specific area of the problem. Palpation helps in assessing the level of tenderness and the active and passive range of motion of the affected joint or joints. To assess active range, the doctor will ask you to move the affected joint or body parts through a specific range of motion. Then you will relax, and the physician will move or assist you to move the affected parts through the same range of motion. The nature and circumstances of any tenderness, swelling, or limitation of the range of motion provide specific diagnostic clues.

DIAGNOSIS

The complete history, examination, and assessment of your complaint enables the physician to determine the probable nature of your joint problem. You may have one or more of the following.

- A soft-tissue abnormality, such as problems with ligaments, tendons, or muscles
- Non-inflammatory arthritis, such as osteoarthritis
- Inflammatory arthritis, such as rheumatoid arthritis

In making such determinations, the physician is guided by training in diagnostic criteria and guidelines and by experience. For the diagnosis of osteoarthritis, for example, the American College of Rheumatology, the premier medical organization in the field of osteoarthritis, has established specific criteria for the classification and diagnosis of osteoarthritis in various joints. Based on extensive scientific evidence, these criteria rely on the findings of the medical history, physical examination, laboratory tests, and radiographic tests (x-rays). If you would like to see the criteria for specific joints, I've included them in the Resources.

WHEN TO SEE A SPECIALIST

Depending on the results of an initial evaluation like that just described, your primary care physician may wish to refer you to a specialist in joint problems. Such specialists include rheumatologists, orthopedists, physical therapists, and occupational therapists. Often these specialists work together as a health care team to provide a range of services that you may need to best treat and rehabilitate an injured or diseased joint. Here's a brief description of each specialty and the type of services and care provided.

Rheumatologists. These medical doctors are internists or pediatricians who have further training in diagnosing and treating diseases of the joints, muscles, bones, and connective tissue. They are also usually board-certified, which means that they have passed very rigorous exams conducted by the American Board of Internal Medicine. Rheumatologists treat all forms of arthritis, certain autoimmune diseases, and other disorders related to the joints, bones, muscles, or connective tissue—more than 100 in all. Many of these diseases are disabling and sometimes fatal; many are complicated and hard to treat. Some of the more common diseases of this type include osteoarthritis, rheumatoid arthritis, lupus, osteoporosis, Lyme disease, fibromylagia, carpal tunnel syndrome, and gout.

Orthopedists. These medical doctors are surgeons who have advanced training in the working and treatment of the musculoskeletal system. Orthopedic surgeons are board-certified after passing rigorous examinations given by the American Board of Orthopaedic Surgery. They diagnose, treat, and rehabilitate injuries and disorders of the muscles, bones, joints, ligaments, tendons, and nerves. They perform surgery for joint repair and joint replacement. Beyond general orthopedics, some orthopedists may further specialize in treating particular joints, such as knees, hips, hands, and shoulders, or in other aspects of orthopedics, such as trauma or sports medicine.

Physical therapists. These professionals are not medical doctors, but they are specially trained in the prevention and rehabilitation of injuries and disorders of the musculoskeletal system. Most have master's degrees. A physical therapist will initially assess how much your joint problem, such as arthritis or a knee injury, is affecting your daily life and what limitations you have. The therapist will then help you improve your function by assisting you in muscle-strengthening and range-of-motion exercises.

Occupational therapists. Although sometimes confused with physical therapists, these professionals are specially trained to help people achieve independence in all aspects of their lives. People who face challenges due to arthritis and other joint problems are just one of the groups they work with. Occupational therapists are specifically trained to evaluate environments, to recommend adaptations and adaptive equipment to help you achieve the highest performance possible, and, in general, to help you function to the very best of your ability in every normal setting, whether at work, at home, or in recreational activities.

SPECIALIZED TESTS AND EVALUATIONS

In addition to standard physical examinations, your physician or specialist in joint health has a number of other diagnostic techniques available to help identify the cause of joint problems and determine proper therapy. Here are some of the most common.

X-rays. Radiographic imagery (as x-rays are called in scientific lingo) has been a valuable tool for diagnosing joint problems for several decades. It was the first of our modern, high-tech diagnostic arsenal. Criteria for using x-rays for diagnosis were first established in 1957 and are still in use today. This diagnostic technique allows the physician to see changes in the joint compartment. The radiographic image reflects the internal structures of the joint—soft tissue, bone density, and space within the joint. With this information, the doctor can analyze various aspects of joint structure, such as the thickness and state of the cartilage pad, the condition of the bone behind the articular cartilage, and so on. To get the best images, your joint will often be x-rayed from several angles.

Computerized tomography (CT) scan. Often called a cat scan, the CT scan is an x-ray that's gone high-tech. The CT equipment combines x-rays with computer imaging to produce a highly accurate, detailed, cross-sectional picture of structures inside the body in relation to other internal structures. CT scans may be used especially in diagnosis of lower-back problems. CT arthrography is a variation of the CT scan that is often used in diagnosing shoulder problems

Magnetic resonance imaging (MRI). MRI is a very effective diagnostic scanning tool that produces cross-sectional images of structures within the body. Unlike the CT scan, MRI technology uses magnetic fields (radio waves created by large rotating magnets), not radiation, to create the images, so there is no risk of harmful exposure. Because MRI has the ability to display anatomy and any pathological changes with better definition and detail than x-ray imaging techniques, it offers high sensitivity to early pathological changes, which makes early detection possible. Physicians often select MRI to help diagnose torn knee cartilage and ligaments, herniated disks in the spine, hip problems, and similar problems.

Ultrasound imaging. Ultrasound technology bounces very high frequency sound waves off the body's internal structures to create an image of their size, shape, location, or composition. Like MRI, ultrasound uses no radiation.

CREATING PARTNERSHIPS FOR CARE

Over the years, I have come to believe strongly that the best medical care results from partnerships between patients and physicians. By understanding how medical evaluation can assist in keeping your joints healthy and how certain evaluations and techniques can help diagnose problems in their earliest stages, you can be an informed patient-partner, ready to work with your physician to devise the best procedures to keep your joints healthy so you can have an active, independent life.

Medications and Other Treatments for Joint Problems

From the over-the-counter pain reliever you take for a mild ache in a joint to the latest joint replacement surgery, the many medications and other therapies for joint problems present a bewildering array of choices. The following overview of the most common treatments for joint pain due to typical injury or osteoarthritis is intended to help you be a better-informed partner with your physician.

A note about inflammatory arthritis: Because rheumatoid arthritis and other inflammatory arthritic diseases—and their treatments—are complex and vary greatly from person to person, I do not address typical therapies for those disorders here. Of course, the broader principles of patient education and participation in therapy and of combining drug therapies with other modes of therapy apply to all joint problems.

SELF-TREATMENT WITH OTC PAIN RELIEVERS

When a joint begins to ache, perhaps after a day of working in the yard or maybe for no reason at all, most people usually self-treat the problem with an over-the-counter painkiller. The product that physicians recommend trying first for relief is acetaminophen, which is the primary ingredient in Tylenol, Anacin-3, Panadol, and other products. A typical dose is 325 to 650 milligrams every 4 to 6 hours as needed. Some timed-release medications are effective for 8 hours so that you can sleep uninterrupted by pain.

Although acetaminophen at recommended levels has few immediate side effects for most adults, long-term use can increase your risk of kidney disease or liver damage. Many adverse side effects can also occur if acetaminophen is used with alcohol or other drugs. Also, while caffeine may enhance the short-term pain-relieving effect, it may decrease long-term pain relief by increasing your tolerance to the drug so that the usual dose is not as effective. As always, if pain lasts for more than 24 hours, see your doctor for further assessment of your problem.

Instead of acetaminophen, many people reach first for an over-the-counter nonsteroidal anti-inflammatory drug (NSAID), such as ibuprofen or naproxen. See the following section on anti-inflammatories for more about NSAIDs.

PATIENT EDUCATION

If your joint pain is more serious or more persistent than an occasional twinge, you should consult your doctor for a diagnosis and proper treatment. After your health care provider has diagnosed your joint problem, education about your specific disease is an extremely important part of any course of treatment. Your physician may give you various pamphlets and direct you to resources available via the mail or online from organizations such as the Arthritis Foundation. See the Resources for sources of educational materials and other information.

In addition, your physician will outline the appropriate treatment for your problem. Many of us who were born or reached maturity in the second half of the 20th century are accustomed not only to a fast-paced society but also to the wonders of modern drugs and surgery. Consequently, we tend to want quick fixes for joint problems—the latest wonder drug, please. However, for mild or moderate osteoarthritis, for joint injuries that don't require immediate surgery, and for rehabilitation after surgery, physicians most often prescribe as the core therapy many of the lifestyle methods emphasized in the 8-Week Joint Health Program. These include but are not limited to aerobic exercise; muscle-strengthening exercise; physical therapy to develop flexibility and range of motion; weight loss, if necessary; and sound nutrition. The doctor will also prescribe pain medications, such as those discussed below, in support of these core "nonpharmacologic modalities."

THE ANTI-INFLAMMATORIES

There are three categories of anti-inflammatory medications for treating joint problems: NSAIDs, steroid medications, and disease-modifying anti-rheumatic drugs (DMARDs). In some cases where pain is severe and does not respond to these therapies, a physician may temporarily use stronger pain relievers, but they are not generally part of standard, long-term drug therapy.

NSAIDs. These medications constitute the most common treatment for several joint problems, including osteoarthritis, even though the inflammation in osteoarthritis is primarily localized and not severe. NSAIDs are most effective when pain is accompanied by inflammation, because the drugs act by inhibiting prostaglandins, the substances that trigger inflammation and pain. The most common NSAIDs include aspirin, ibuprofen (Motrin, Advil, Nuprin), naproxen (Aleve, Anaprox), and ketoprofen (Orudis, Oruvail, Actron). There is no clear evidence, however, that one type works better than others for the pain of osteoarthritis. Because the dosage of different NSAIDs varies greatly, follow the manufacturer's and your physician's recommendations. If you are taking an over-the-counter NSAID, never exceed the recommended dosage.

Although many people use NSAIDs for long-term treatment, most of these drugs have side effects, particularly stomach discomfort and other gastric disorders, that tend to be more common the longer the drug is taken. There can also be other side effects, depending on the specific drug. Taking NSAIDs with food has been shown to reduce gastric problems, but this can also slow pain relief. Long-term use can damage the stomach, possibly causing ulcers and gastrointestinal bleeding (buffering the drugs with an antacid is not effective in reducing this risk). Older adults, smokers, and people who consume alcohol are more likely to experience these problems. NSAIDs may also increase the risk of elevated blood pressure, especially for people already diagnosed with hypertension, and of dizziness, ringing in the ears, headache, skin rash, and possibly depression. Long-term treatment with these medications should be done only with the supervision of a physician.

Steroid medications. If your pain is severe and you also have inflammation, your physician may prescribe corticosteroid injections. Steroid treatment should be used with great caution because it masks pain and does not reduce cartilage deterioration from either osteoarthritis or an injured joint. You should have no more than three corticosteroid shots per year, because the drugs can cause many potentially serious side effects that affect the central nervous and cardiovascular systems as well as the eyes and endocrine system.

DMARDs. These drugs can slow the disease process in many joint conditions. Because they may take 6 to 8 months to produce a noticeable effect, they are used if NSAIDs and other painkillers fail to provide relief. They are known to be especially effective for people with rheumatoid arthritis because they control synovial inflammation. They are also used for ankylosing spondylitis, psoriatic arthritis, and lupus.

PHYSICAL THERAPY

Physical therapy includes the use of heat and ice treatments, range-of-motion and strengthening exercises, and ultrasound treatment directed by a physical therapist or other health care professional. A major objective of much physical therapy is to strengthen the muscles around the affected joint in order to protect it from repetitive trauma that can accelerate wear.

PROTECTIVE AND ASSISTIVE DEVICES

If you have a joint injury, perhaps a sprain or strain, your physician may prescribe and fit you with a cast, splint, or brace to protect the joint. Your doctor may also advise using a cane, crutches, or other assistive devices for either injury or to help relieve osteoarthritis.

SURGICAL INTERVENTION

Although surgery is always a last resort, it may be required or recommended in some cases to prevent further physical damage not only to the joint but also to the musculoskeletal system as a whole. A joint injury, including the degenerative effects of osteoarthritis, can cause other bones and muscles to overcompensate to make up for areas of weakness. Some traumatic injuries, such as totally ruptured ligaments or tendons, may require immediate surgery to restore function to the joint. Depending on the nature of the problem, joint surgery can be as simple as the removal of small pieces of bone or cartilage or as serious as total joint replacement.

NEW AND EMERGING THERAPIES

Recently, the new NSAIDs celecoxib (Celebrex) and rofecoxib (Vioxx) have become available. The benefit that these drugs offer over other NSAIDS is that they may protect against gastrointestinal side effects because they block only the prostaglandin-producing enzyme called cyclooxygenase 2 (COX 2). They allow the body to continue to produce the enzyme cyclooxygenase 1 (COX 1), which stimulates the prostaglandins that protect the stomach. These drugs have become so popular among physicians that they are now among the most commonly prescribed medications for joint problems.

Among new therapies for the knee, the most common site of joint pain, a new injection therapy called visco supplementation shows promise for patients who do not respond well to the use of NSAIDs and a program of lifestyle therapy. In this procedure, fluid is drained from the inflamed knee and replaced with hyaluronic acid (Synvisc, Hyalgan), a natural substance that the body uses to lubricate the joints. The mechanism of this therapy is not yet clearly understood, but among other actions, hyaluronic acid may fight inflammation and stimulate the growth of new cartilage cells.

A SOUND APPROACH TO THERAPY

As you see, although medications alone don't hold the answer to overcoming joint pain, when used under the direction of your physician and in conjunction with other therapies, they can provide both substantial relief from pain and improvement in function. Often, not having to deal with pain means that you can comfortably pursue the therapeutic exercises and physical activities that are so important to long-term improvement.

Alternative Therapies

In the United States, the past 10 to 15 years have seen a surge of interest in what is known as alternative medicine or, increasingly, as complementary medicine. An estimated one-third or more of the U.S. population participates to some degree in various therapies that have been lumped together under these designations. Pain, particularly chronic pain, is a major reason that many people seek alternative therapy. Those who have joint pain, therefore, may have a particular interest in exploring alternative therapies to either supplement or replace some traditional medical therapies.

Although many of the therapies that have been clustered under the rubric of "alternative therapy" may have some merit, at the other end of a wide spectrum are so-called therapies that are merely hype at best and dangerous at worst. Evaluating alternative therapies that may have value for you requires caution, common sense, and good judgment. The following information will help you separate fact from fiction.

ALTERNATIVE THERAPY VERSUS LIFESTYLE MEDICINE

Although there are many definitions of alternative medicine (in fact, that's part of the difficulty), most people would consider "unconventional" therapies or therapies not generally used in Western medicine as alternative. The daily lifestyle practices recommended in this book to promote joint health are alternative therapy in a different sense: They give you a positive alternative to developing the joint pain and arthritis that typically come with aging.

I like to view this branch of medicine as lifestyle medicine. By this I mean those practices in our daily lives that can have a major impact on our health. These may be physical activity, proper nutrition, weight management, or even supplementation. In all of these instances, significant, good studies confirm the benefits of taking these simple steps to improve our health.

In addition to lifestyle medicine and the conventional therapies of Western medicine, you may wish to consider which of a number of additional or alternative therapies may offer some truly complementary benefits.

MIND/BODY TECHNIQUES AND SPIRITUALITY

There is no question that there are profound links between mind and body. In fact, a number of studies of people with arthritis have looked at how someone responds to pain as a very important consideration in therapy. At my laboratory, we have conducted a number of studies examining the interaction between mind and body. Such studies show that techniques such as visualization, meditation, the "relaxation response," and many others may have a profound effect on how each of us deals with the pain of joint problems and other conditions. In any large city, you can find opportunities to try meditation, biofeedback, visualization, or other mind/body techniques. I believe that these techniques can have tremendous positive impact on the management of chronic conditions such as arthritis, and I strongly encourage you to explore some of these options.

Recently, some investigators have focused their attention on spirituality as one form of mind/body technique for treating conditions such as chronic pain. Spirituality, in this sense, does not necessarily mean formal religion but refers to techniques that involve a consciousness of your spiritual well-being. Findings to date suggest that such techniques can have a very important impact on managing the chronic pain of joint disease.

ACUPUNCTURE AND ACUPRESSURE

Acupuncture has been used by millions of people around the world to treat many ailments. In the United States, acupuncture is being used increasingly within Western medicine for a variety of conditions, but most prominently for pain relief. Many people think that acupuncture requires inserting needles into the body, but there are related forms of treatment that treat various acupuncture energy points with heat, herbs, or pressure. When pressure is used, the technique is called acupressure.

I believe that acupuncture and acupressure have enormous potential to relieve the symptoms of joint problems. If you are thinking of using either, find a properly trained individual to perform these techniques for you (although one of the advantages of acupressure is that once you have learned the techniques, you can also use them yourself). The best advice is to select practitioners who are certified by the national certifying bodies for these types of therapies. One such organization is the National Certification Commission for Acupuncture and Oriental Medicine, or NCCAOM (703-584-9004; www.nccaom.org). Many medical doctors are now becoming certified in acupuncture. Your family physician may have this certification or be able to refer you to a certified practitioner.

MASSAGE

Massage can also offer many benefits to people who have joint problems and other conditions that cause chronic pain. I am a firm believer in the healing power of touch.

In general terms, massage involves the manipulation of the soft tissue and layers of muscle through pressure, kneading, and stroking. It can employ a wide variety of different techniques. Again, it's important to find a massage therapist who is skilled and careful, particularly if you have existing joint problems. Several national organizations certify massage therapists, including the National Certification Board for Therapeutic Massage and Bodywork (800-296-0664; www.ncbtmb.com) and the American Massage Therapy Association

(847-864-0123; www.amtamassage.org). Both organizations have Web sites with good information, and both can help you find certified massage therapists in your area.

MISCELLANEOUS THERAPIES

Like other chronic pain syndromes, joint pain has given rise to a wide variety of particular therapies, some of which may have some benefit and some of which, in my opinion, carry no benefit at all. Let's explore two of the most popular.

Magnet therapy. Magnets have been around for centuries, and claims for their healing benefits have been around for almost as long. Although magnets used to create a microwave field in MRI equipment certainly help us get a better diagnostic view of joint problems, there is not currently enough information to make a firm recommendation about magnet therapy. We need further research in this area. If you do want to try magnet therapy, I'd advise you to make a small investment in magnets and ask for a money-back guarantee before you purchase any of this type of equipment.

Copper bracelets. A lot of folklore and anecdotal reports support the use of copper bracelets to control arthritis pain. But, at this point, the medical literature does not support this claim. I would be very cautious about attributing healing powers to wearing a copper bracelet.

Part of the apparent pain-relieving power of copper in some people may result from the placebo effect. Because the mind is truly powerful, if you actually think that you are going to improve, sometimes you do. This effect is not negative; it's just a part of human psychology. In scientific studies, in fact, the placebo effect can account for up to a 30 percent difference in results. That is why, in any major medical study, we have a control group that receives placebos. In order for the substance being tested to be judged effective, the group receiving that active substance has to have a higher percentage of positive results than could be attributed to the expected placebo effect. It is only through this kind of rigorous trial that we can really show whether a practice or a therapy has benefits. At this point, there have been no such trials to test the efficacy of copper bracelets to relieve pain.

ALTERNATIVE HEALING AND BELIEF SYSTEMS

Of course, as a practitioner of Western medicine, I have received extensive training in the thought patterns that underlie it. This is not to say that other forms and belief systems that comprise healing systems are not also valid. People who have chronic pain often will seek advice from a wide variety of laypeople and practitioners who have different healing belief systems. Let's look at a few of these.

Chiropractic. Chiropractic, the third-largest health care profession in this country, is used by more than 50 million Americans each year. Most people go to chiropractors for treatment of back or neck pain following an injury or an accident. Many of my patients have told me that they have achieved great benefits for musculoskeletal problems from visits to chiropractors.

There are 17 accredited chiropractic colleges in the United States, where chiropractors complete a 4-year program. The key is finding a practitioner of chiropractic whom you like and have confidence in. Chiropractors are licensed in all states; I recommend that if you are interested in chiropractic treatment, you find a member of the American Chiropractic Association (800-986-4636; www.amerchiro.org). Because many physicians are now working with chiropractors in treating musculoskeletal problems, your physician may be able to refer you to a good chiropractor.

Osteopathic medicine. Doctors of osteopathy (whose professional degree is D.O.) complete professional training that is very similar to that of medical doctors (M.D.'s). I have had the pleasure of working with many osteopathic doctors and have found them to be highly competent, with thought patterns and backgrounds that are similar to those of M.D.'s. Osteopathy as a profession emphasizes the healing touch—literally, hands-on medicine—which is an approach that many people with joint pain may find beneficial.

Once again, if you are thinking about receiving therapy from a doctor of osteopathy, it is important that you find someone who is well-regarded and certified. The certifying organization is the American Osteopathic Association (800-621-1773; www.aoa-net.org).

Chinese medicine. Chinese medicine has been practiced for thousands of years. Increasingly, it is being used in the United States, often in conjunction with traditional Western medicine. The key principles of Chinese medicine involve balancing energy and vital life force, which is called *qi* (pronounced *chee*). Acupuncture is one of many therapeutic techniques in the larger philosophy and practice of Chinese medicine, and the gentle, flowing exercise of tai chi, another technique associated with Chinese medicine, is an excellent physical activity for people with joint pain and stiffness such as that caused by osteoarthritis. Some of my patients have achieved a great deal of benefit from this modality. You can locate a practitioner of Chinese medicine by getting in touch with the American Association of Oriental Medicine (888-500-7999; www.aaom.org). The NCCAOM (see page 158) can also help you locate a certified practitioner.

WORKING WITH YOUR PHYSICIAN

Although you may find some benefits from various alternative therapies, I strongly urge you to discuss any of them with your physician. I have always been troubled by the fact that 75 percent of people who use alternative medicine never discuss it with their regular physicians. I feel that this is a mistake because as we in Western medicine are opening our hearts and minds to some of the unconventional therapies, it is important for our patients to communicate with us about the alternative therapies that they are pursuing. This is particularly vital because some of these therapies may interact in very significant ways with therapies and medications prescribed by traditional physicians. My best advice to you is that if you are seeking treatment with alternative therapies, use them in conjunction with traditional medicine, not to the exclusion of it. Make it truly *complementary* medicine.

Keeping Your Joints Young

We all want to live to a ripe old age and have the final years of life be full of enjoyment, free of pain, and complete with the "prize" that comes from a lifetime of healthy living. We also want to function at our best and not be limited or dependent on other people any more than is humanly possible.

Make no mistake, the health of your joints is critically important to a healthy and fulfilling old age. In fact, joint health is inextricably linked to overall good health. You simply cannot have one without the other. People who have problems with their joints become increasingly inactive, which triggers a number of problems. Inactivity dramatically increases the risk of heart disease, diabetes, other chronic diseases, and obesity. Quality of life plummets. In fact, inactivity sets up a vicious cycle: The more inactive people become, the more weight they gain. The more weight they gain, the more joint problems they have. The more joint problems, the less activity, and so on in a downward spiral. Their muscles become weaker and their joints and muscles become even stiffer, compounding the problem. Almost inevitably, osteoarthritis attacks and then worsens.

Although aging is a proven risk factor for joint problems, they are not an inevitable part of the aging process. Actions that you can take today and adopt throughout life can have a profound, positive impact on whether you will have joint problems in your later years. The good news in all of this is that it is never too late to start. Even people in their sixties and seventies can benefit from the advice that I have given throughout this book about how to adopt the habits that will improve joint health and promote overall good health.

THE EFFECTS OF AGING

As I have said, your joints are complex and wonderfully adaptive. Many components must work properly in order for a joint to be healthy, and all of these components, to some degree, are susceptible to changes related to aging. Muscles may become less strong and pliable as we age, for example. Also, bones and cartilage have a tendency to thin out and wear away, particularly in weight-bearing joints. Furthermore, a lifetime of wear and tear on the joints can result in cumulative problems that begin to manifest themselves as you age. It is no wonder that more than 20 percent of people over age 70 have significant osteoarthritis of one or both knees.

Fortunately, many of these aging processes can be significantly slowed. In fact, a number of studies have shown that a lifetime of practicing good nutrition, being physically active, and maintaining a healthy weight will slow the decline in virtually every physiologic function. Thus, while you can't stop the passage of years, you can kick aging in the seat of the pants. Most studies have shown that physically active people keep good physiological function three times longer than inactive people do.

AGING AND GENERAL HEALTH

Of course, joints are not the only body system that's affected by aging. It touches the cardiovascular system, muscular system, and virtually every other biological system in the body. A number of studies have shown, however, that people who take charge of their health from an early age can slow the aging process in very dramatic ways. While I am not saying that we have discovered the Fountain of Youth, it's true that our daily actions can alter the aging process significantly.

I like to tell my patients that each of us has three ages: our chronological age, our physiological age, and our spiritual age. We can't do anything about our chronological age; it simply numbers the years that we have been on the planet. We can take charge of our physiological age, however. We all know people who have not taken good care of themselves and who look and act much older than they are. But guess what? You can look and act *younger* than you are. The same steps that benefit joint health can ensure that your physiological age stays younger than your actual years. I know an 82-year-old who's still running down the drive to catch the mail truck or up the stairs to answer the phone. That's going to be me—and it can be you, too.

Part of the key also lies in our "spiritual" age, which too many people forget about. Most of us know people who are lively and vital and inquisitive into their eighties and nineties. They have spiritually refused to grow old. They always look for new challenges and ask questions that inspire everyone around them to act and think young. So, physiologically and spiritually at least, we can keep the negative effects of aging at bay.

CONTROLLING SYMPTOMS AND MAINTAINING FUNCTION

As we age, two major considerations that we face are how to minimize joint pain and how to maximize joint function. The good news is that the program described in this book works for a lifetime to help you prevent joint problems, slow the progress of osteoarthritis, and reduce symptoms of existing problems. It's also never too late to start the program. Of course, in some instances, medications such as those discussed in chapter 13 can be extremely beneficial. Furthermore, taking supplements (see chapter 10) can have an enormous positive impact on controlling pain and improving function, just as it did for the subjects in our research study.

TIPS FOR LIFETIME JOINT HEALTH

All of the recommendations in the 8-Week Joint Health Program can be used by people in their sixties, seventies, and beyond. There are a few instances in which people need to exercise particular caution, however, and I note these as necessary.

Establish a walking program. Walking is the ideal exercise for older people to maintain both good cardiovascular health and joint health. In studies conducted at my laboratory, many people in their seventies and eighties participate in walking programs, both for general good health and to lower their risk of various chronic diseases, lose weight, and improve their joint health. I strongly recommend that older people who are starting a walking program get a pair of good, well-cushioned walking shoes. Because it is important to get good foot care, a visit to a podiatrist is also worthwhile.

Of course, if you already have joint problems, you should always check with your physician before beginning any program. The combination of walking and taking appropriate anti-inflammatory agents and/or supplements can go a long way toward helping you to control the symptoms of osteoarthritis and other joint problems. Sometimes, getting started and then persevering through the first few weeks of becoming more active is the hardest part. So commit for the long haul, and you will usually realize the benefits.

Increase other physical activity. Of all of the recommendations that I make to my older patients, perhaps the one that comes up most often is "Stay active!" For people in their seventies and eighties, physical activity not only is important for joint health and cardiovascular health, it is particularly important for balance, since balance problems can result in falls that cause disastrous injuries and the end of independent living. In one study at my institute, in which we tested more than 340 people between the ages of 40 and 80, we found that the level of physical activity was the single best predictor for how good a person's balance was. So if you want to have a healthy old age, be sure that you have an *active* old age.

Pursue strength training and stretching. Strong muscles are less likely to be injured. Muscles and joints that are put through a regular stretching program are much more likely to be healthy, well-nourished, and limber. The strength-training and stretching programs and recommendations in chapter 7 are designed to be appropriate for people of all ages. The tests in chapter 4 will help you start at the right level for your present condition.

A number of studies have shown that older people, even in their eighties and nineties, can significantly improve their strength through a structured strength-training program. If you are over 70, however, I strongly recommend that you seek advice from a certified athletic trainer or a physical therapist to help you establish a good program that will work safely for you. Using such professional help is particularly important if you have any existing joint problems.

Work on weight management. Maintaining proper weight throughout life, and particularly after the age of 60, is vitally important to joint health. Carrying excess weight not only creates extra pounding and stress on the joints, it is also thought to trigger the release of hormones that may contribute to the breakdown of cartilage and other joint structures. Weight management is one of the first things that I discuss with overweight people in their sixties and seventies.

Achieve proper nutrition. Good nutrition is important at any stage of life, but it is absolutely vital after age 60. Many older people have a particular challenge in maintaining good nutrition. Often, it is inconvenient and difficult for them to chop or otherwise prepare food, but the effort is worth it. Having adequate calcium in the diet for bone health, eating at least five servings of fruits and vegetables a day, and other nutritionally sound practices, as presented in chapter 9, are all vitally important.

In addition, the Framingham Osteoarthritis Study found that people who had adequate intakes of vitamin C were one-third as likely to develop osteoarthritis as those who did not get enough. Another interesting finding from that study is that people who had proper levels of vitamin D (available from fortified low-fat milk products, among other sources) had a much slower progression of joint problems than people who did not maintain adequate levels. One good practice that I recommend if you are over age 60 is to see a registered dietitian to discuss specific nutritional concerns related to both joint health and overall good health.

Consider mind/body connections. As already discussed, issues relating to the interaction of mind and body are very important to many aspects of good health, and particularly to joint health. People who have chronic joint pain can often lapse into depression and experience a poor quality of life. Numerous studies have also shown that people who are depressed tend to have more difficulty with the painful symptoms of osteoarthritis and other joint problems. Remember that mind and body are inextricably linked. Maintaining a positive attitude to go with an active lifestyle can be a key to staying healthy in your older years and having a high quality of life throughout a lifetime. If you are feeling depressed, don't hesitate to discuss it with your physician, who has a number of options to help you deal with the problem.

Use supplementation as appropriate. I believe that the findings of our research study are particularly relevant as people age. Remember that the subjects recruited for the study were between the ages of 40 and 80. People in their sixties, seventies, and eighties frequently have difficulty obtaining all the proper nutrients from their diets. They are also often taking various medications. When taking a supplement such as most of those discussed in chapter 10, it is unlikely that you will have any interactions with any of the drugs that you may be taking for medical problems. Furthermore, the substances found in gelatin-based supplements (gelatin, vitamin C, vitamin D, calcium, and other minerals) are all very important as we age. Supplementation is an easy and safe way for older people to enhance joint health. Just remember to tell your physician about any supplementation that you choose.

A WORKING PARTNERSHIP

If you are over age 60, I think it is particularly important to work with your physician to establish specific plans for good joint health and overall health. Because older people are more likely to experience adverse interactions among various medicines, in addition to facing other problems associated with aging, it is very important to establish a comfortable working relationship with your physician.

CHOOSE TO BE HEALTHY

None of us will live forever, but all of us should strive to make our time on this planet as happy and healthy as possible. Our views of healthy aging have changed dramatically over the past few years. It is now abundantly clear from many studies that a good many of what we used to regard as inevitable problems of aging are really related to a progressively sedentary lifestyle and the societal expectations that the older we get, the less active we should be. Let's turn that around. Let's adopt lifestyles that are active and healthy. This is the best way to combat joint problems as we age, and certainly to promote healthy, pain-free joints for an active, fulfilling life.

Sports and Joint Health

I want to start this chapter with a confession: I am an avid athlete. Former President George Bush once said that he never met a sport he didn't like. Almost the same could be said of me. In addition to my personal passion for sports, however, I am also passionate about encouraging everyone to become more physically active. The enjoyment and multiple health benefits that come from sports can benefit everyone.

Although I enthusiastically advocate sports, I also recognize that they can be a source of injury and multiple problems for your joints. In fact, prior injuries (including sports injuries) are the leading cause of osteoarthritis in men. We can change this picture. There are many ways to maximize the health benefits and pure enjoyment of playing recreational sports while minimizing the likelihood of damaging your joints. In fact, when it's done right, regular participation in sports is one of the very best ways I know to promote joint health. Here are the key issues and precautions that you need to consider in order to get these important benefits while participating safely in all sports, from recreational to high-level competitive types.

A NATION OF SPORTS ENTHUSIASTS

Americans love sports. And although, as you know, I am concerned that as a nation we are not active enough, many people participate at least occasionally in sports. In fact, one Neilson survey indicated that almost 600 million people participate annually in sports in the United States.

That figure means that many of us participate in multiple sports. Specifically, swimming, bicycling, walking, and jogging and running lead the way in popularity. Competitive sports, such as tennis, basketball, baseball, and football, also have plenty of participants and offer wonderful ways to enjoy activity and get multiple health benefits.

Unfortunately, sports are also a significant cause of joint injuries. In fact, according to the Consumer Product Safety Council, more than 11 million people each year are injured as a result of either fitness activities or competitive sports. We also know some details about these injuries. First, more than half occur in four sports—bicycling, baseball, football, and basketball. Second, almost three-quarters occur in athletes between the ages of 10 and 24. Third, the most common types of sports injuries include sprains, strains, scrapes, and cuts. Broken bones account for less than 20 percent of all sports injuries.

We also know which joints are most likely to be injured. Fingers and hands lead the list, but different injuries occur in different sports. In basketball, for example, ankle sprains are by far the most frequent injuries, while injuries to the face and head are the most common in bicycling. Both baseball and football are most likely to result in injuries to the fingers and hands, while knee injuries take second place in football.

We have also learned a great deal about how to prevent sports injuries, and that is a major focus of this chapter. One of the key steps is to separate myth from reality.

SPORTS MYTHS

Someone once said that we are a nation of storytellers, and myths definitely can play a powerful role in inspiring us and pointing us toward underlying truths or high ideals. When it comes to sports, however, myths are not good. In fact, many sports myths prevent people from making the right choices to take proper care of their joints. Here are some of the prevalent myths related to joint health and sports.

Myth #1: Fitness walking and running will lead to arthritis in the ankles and knees. There is absolutely no scientific evidence for this. In fact, people who are involved in regular fitness activities are less likely to develop osteoarthritis than those who are not physically active. (See page 173 for more information on this point.) The principal negative consequence of this myth is that it discourages people from becoming more active. Regular physical activity is good for virtually every system of the body, including your joints.

Myth #2: Women are more prone to injury than men. Once again, there is no medical basis for this myth. Over the past 15 to 20 years, as women have become more involved in high-level competition, there was some initial concern that they were experiencing more injuries. Over the past decade, however, these differences have been largely eliminated. Any previous higher injury rate among women, experts suggest, may have occurred because early female competitors often did not have the same level of coaching as men or, in some instances, the same level of conditioning.

Myth #3: Inflammation is bad. Although I noted previously that osteoarthritis has an inflammatory component, I do not want to leave the impression that all inflammation is bad. Actually, the inflammatory process is the body's way of healing itself. The redness, swelling, and other signs associated with inflammation signal that the body has called white blood cells to the injury to fight off infection and clean up waste products, a vital process in healing. When the inflammation becomes chronic, however, it can be self-defeating. That danger is another reason to have injuries treated promptly and follow the doctor's prescription for rehabilitation and rate of return to activity.

Myth #4: You can play yourself into shape after an injury. How often have you heard a sports commentator talk about an athlete "playing himself into shape"? This is a very dangerous myth because pursuing the same activity that caused an injury can prevent total healing. Sports medicine doctors like to talk about the 95 percent rule, meaning that the injury must be 95 percent healed before you can return to the sport. If you pay close attention to this rule, you will minimize the likelihood that an acute injury will turn into a chronic problem.

ARE THERE ANY "SAFE" SPORTS?

The sad truth is that no sporting activity is entirely safe—but neither is getting out of bed. Happily, there are many sports that are comparatively safe. One of the reasons that I am so enthusiastic about walking is that it has such a low injury potential. Of course, you can injure yourself while walking, but the likelihood is much lower than in a higher-impact activity such as running, and certainly lower than in contact sports such as football.

When you think about choosing a safe sport, think about those that cause low impact and ones for which you have basic skills. For example, you can seriously injure yourself even in a "safe" sport such as golf if you have bad biomechanics and put your back, shoulder, or elbow in an unnatural position. Another key is to maintain proper conditioning so that you don't ask your muscles and joints to perform activities that they are not in shape to perform. Proper equipment is also very important to maximize safety. See page 173 for details about preventing injuries.

COMMON JOINT INJURIES

While a variety of joint injuries can occur in sports, there are five that are particularly common: sprains, strains, dislocations, fractures, and degenerative injuries.

Sprains. A sprained ankle is one of the most common injuries. It occurs when the anklebone is forced out of the ankle joint as the ankle is tipped inward or outward. The actual injury in a sprain is the stretching of the ligaments on the outer or inner part of the ankle. Physicians classify sprains as Grade I, Grade II, or Grade III, based on how much the ligaments have been stretched and damaged. If they are stretched only a little, it is a Grade I sprain. If there is a partial tear of the ligament, it is Grade II. A Grade III sprain occurs when the ligament tears completely. Unless your ankle is only mildly "turned," I always recommend that you see a qualified physician to assess the level of sprain. If you don't, you risk turning an acute injury into a chronic one. The same advice goes for other sprains, such as those of the wrists, knees, shoulders, and, yes, even the fingers.

Strains. Strains occur in muscles rather than in joints. Tennis elbow, hamstring pulls, and most shinsplints are all examples of strains. Because strains to a muscle can clearly affect the stability of a joint, it is important to discuss them in the context of sports injuries. Physicians grade muscle strains by the same classifications as sprains. The extent of a muscle strain is determined by how many muscle fibers are actually torn. In a mild strain (Grade I), only a few fibers are torn, whereas in a very significant strain (Grade III), the muscle is completely torn. In each of these instances, the severity of the tear determines the amount of time required for recovery. Grade I strains may heal largely without medical intervention, while Grade II and Grade III strains require medical therapy. Again, see your physician promptly for anything more severe than a mild strain.

Dislocations. A dislocation occurs when one of the bones in a joint is actually pulled out of it. Usually, a dislocation requires immediate attention from a qualified medical practitioner to return the bone to the joint and then stabilize it. The shoulder joint is most susceptible because of the wide range of activities that it performs and the resulting range of motion that it must go through. The shoulder also plays an important role in the motions required in many sports, from baseball to skiing.

Fractures. There are two basic types of fractures, a complete fracture, in which the bone is broken completely through, and a stress fracture, in which the bone is cracked but not separated. With a few minor exceptions, fractures require prompt medical therapy and will often require immobilization, such as the use of a cast.

Degenerative injuries. Degenerative injuries occur from repeated trauma over a period of years. Professional football linemen, for example, often have degenerative injuries in their knees because they have to carry a lot of body weight and move rapidly and repeatedly up and down in a squatting position. Improperly treated sports injuries (such as returning to a sport too soon and too often after injuries) can also lead to degenerative changes, such as those of osteoarthritis.

PRINCIPLES OF TREATMENT

The principles of immediate treatment for sprains and strains can be described by the acronym RICE, which stands for rest, ice, compression, and elevation. If you have an ankle sprain, for example, you should immediately stop walking or running on it, then apply ice as quickly as possible. Once the swelling has gone down, using compression with an Ace bandage is worthwhile. Elevating the leg will also minimize swelling. If you have any injury that you think is more than a mild sprain or strain, though, you should seek immediate medical attention.

CAN SPORTS LEAD TO OSTEOARTHRITIS?

As I said in the discussion of the myths of sports, the bottom line is that, compared with sedentary people, those who are involved in regular physical activity such as fitness walking or jogging significantly minimize their risk of developing osteoarthritis. In fact, the rate of osteoarthritis in regular walkers or runners is only about 2 percent.

There are certain situations, however, in which osteoarthritis may occur in people who play sports consistently throughout their lifetimes. First, improperly treated sports injuries can lead to osteoarthritis farther down the road, particularly if the same joint is injured repeatedly. Second, people who participate in sports that involve repetitive pounding and a high potential for injury may also have an increased incidence of osteoarthritis. Studies have shown that athletes who participate in high-level competitive sports such as soccer or football throughout their sports careers also have a higher rate of osteoarthritis. Also, people such as football linemen or weightlifters who keep their body weights high because of their sports are somewhat predisposed to osteoarthritis. But these situations do not apply to most people, and what I want to emphasize is that recreational physical activity is actually good for joints and not something to fear.

AN OUNCE OF PREVENTION

If you are going to be active as I recommend, in either a fitness program or recreational sports, I think the following basic concepts are important to minimize the risk of injury.

Choose the right activity. As I have already indicated, recreational activities that have low injury potential, such as fitness walking, are very unlikely to cause injuries to the joints. Even if you choose a higher-impact activity, such as running, using proper caution and achieving good conditioning and proper skills can minimize your risk.

Practice physical conditioning. Joints that are used and strong are less likely to be injured or cause problems than joints that are weak from inactivity. The weekend warrior who injures a joint has probably contributed to the likelihood of injury by not keeping his joints in proper condition.

Warm up and cool down properly. I always advocate that you do from 5 to 7 minutes of light exercise and stretching both before starting and after completing an exercise session or a game. Failure to do this can lead to a lot of joint problems.

Choose equipment carefully. Modern equipment has revolutionized sports safety and performance. It is very important to choose well-designed protective equipment that will minimize your risk of injury. This choice can be as simple as selecting a good pair of walking or running shoes or as involved as purchasing proper equipment for downhill skiing or even wind surfing. In addition, although it doesn't offer joint protection, I urge cyclists to select good helmets to wear whenever they bicycle outdoors.

Vary your activities. One of the ways to minimize overuse injuries is to vary sports from season to season. When I play sports in addition to following my fitness program, I tend to select one or two favorite sports each season, stick with them for that season, and then move on to another activity. That's good advice, not only to keep your joints healthy but also to keep your interest and motivation high.

Learn as much as you can. The more you know about a sport and how to participate in it, the less likely you are to be injured. I think that having good coaching is also a key part of educating yourself about how to safely participate in a sport.

WHEN TO SEE A DOCTOR

I am often asked about the circumstances in which people should seek medical treatment for sports injuries. I believe that the best general answer is to use your common sense and err on the side of caution. Any injury to the joint or the muscles related to a joint is reason for a doctor visit. Having a qualified physician evaluate any joint injury usually means that an acute injury will not become a chronic problem. Other symptoms, such as a decrease in function or significant pain, should also cue you to seek medical attention.

THE IMPORTANCE OF REHABILITATION

If you have had a sports injury, I cannot overemphasize the importance of proper rehabilitation. This is where physical therapists typically join with physicians to help you regain function of an injured joint. Too often, people think that they can rehabilitate a joint on their own, but don't make this mistake. Physical therapists are specifically trained to understand the anatomy of a joint and help with the healing process. Such professionals can help you resolve problems with the joint and also build up the muscles around it to encourage a full recovery. Failure to get proper physical therapy is one of the most common reasons for ongoing joint problems.

TOWARD AN ACTIVE, SAFE LIFESTYLE

Throughout this book, I have talked about the important role of lifestyle measures in promoting joint health. Number one on my list is regular physical activity, and I include recreational sports in that category. The advantage of sports is that in addition to all of their health benefits, you get the joy of competition and participation. Following some of the simple concepts in this chapter will benefit your joints, your overall health, and your emotional well-being, while minimizing the risk of the kinds of injuries that can lead to joint problems. So lead an active life, and use these strategies to make it as safe as possible.

Resources

RESOURCES FOR PAIN-FREE, HEALTHY JOINTS

In addition to this book, there are lots of resources to support you in your quest for healthy joints. Whether you live in a city apartment or in a cabin in the woods miles from the nearest town, if you have access to the Internet, reams (or should I say bytes?) of reliable information are just a few clicks away. Many of the most helpful organizations can also be reached by phone, and there are books and other printed materials available as well.

The following are some of the resources that I have found most useful and reliable. Of course, there's much more information out there, but you can use this list as a starting point from which to explore the topics covered in *The Joint Health Prescription*. The list is arranged to correspond with chapter topics and elements in the 8-Week Joint Health Program. In general, resources given in specific chapters are not repeated here.

JOINT HEALTH AND GENERAL HEALTH

If you were to search the Internet for either an aspect of health such as "joint health/disease" or a particular condition such as "osteoarthritis," you would find literally hundreds of Web sites, newsgroups, and chat rooms, not to mention marketers of various products. Here are a few easy-to-use, reputable sites, most of which have links to additional sites. I've included sites related not only to joint health but also to general health and to some of the more common conditions that older people with arthritis may have, such as cardiovascular disease or diabetes. I've also listed some good books on the same topics.

Check out the following sites for sound information about joint health and joint problems, including osteoarthritis and other forms of arthritis.

▧ The American Academy of Orthopaedic Surgeons: http://orthoinfo.aaos.org

■ The American College of Rheumatology: www.rheumatology.org
■ The Arthritis Foundation: www.arthritis.org
■ The Arthritis National Research Foundation:
www.curearthritis.org
■ Johns Hopkins Arthritis: www.hopkins-arthritis.som.jhmi.edu

The following sites offer good, basic information on general health and many specific conditions and diseases.

■ The American Heart Association: www.americanheart.org
■ The American Medical Association: www.ama-assn.org
■ Harvard Health Letters: www.health.harvard.edu
■ Harvard Medical School consumer health information:
www.intelihealth.com
■ Johns Hopkins health information: www.hopkinsmedicine.org
■ The Mayo Clinic: www.mayohealth.org
■ The National Heart, Lung, and Blood Institute: www.nhlbi.nih.gov

If you are looking for a family health reference that provides a good bit of detail about how the body works and how to keep it healthy, along with information on various specific conditions, diseases, therapies, and treatments, the following books are excellent.

■ *Harvard Medical School Family Health Guide*, edited by Anthony L. Komaroff. New York: Simon & Schuster, 1999.
■ *Johns Hopkins Family Health Book,* edited by Michael Klag et al. New York: HarperCollins, 1999.
■ *Mayo Clinic Family Health Book,* edited by David E. Larson. New York: William Morrow, 1990.

FITNESS AND WALKING

You'll find many resources devoted to all types of fitness, from walking to swimming. Here are some helpful Web sites.

■ About.com, senior health: www.seniorhealth.about.com
■ About.com, walking: www.walking.about.com
■ American Volkssport Association: www.ava.org

- Prevention's Walking Club: www.women.com/clubs/walking/
- Rippe Lifestyle Institute: www.rippelifestyle.com

Look for these two good walking books.

- *Fit over Forty,* by James M. Rippe. New York: Quill, 1996.
- *Prevention's Complete Book of Walking,* by Maggie Spilner. Emmaus, Pa.: Rodale, 2000.

OTHER PHYSICAL ACTIVITIES

Starting with the national Shape Up, America, campaign, physical activity has received a major push from many public and private health care organizations and agencies. Thus, there are now a number of good Web sites. Here are some of my favorites on both general activity and gardening.

- The American Heart Association "Just Move" program: www.justmove.org
- *Fine Gardening* magazine: www.taunton.com/fg/
- GardenWeb.com: www.gardenweb.com
- *Horticulture* magazine: www.hortmag.com
- *Organic Gardening* magazine: www.organicgardening.com
- Utah's physical activity and fitness site: www.utahfitness.org/ugchpf/homepa.html

STRETCHING

Here are two good books about stretching, taking your stretching program further, and learning stretches for specific activities and sports.

- *Book of Body Maintenance and Repair,* by Marilyn Moffat and Steve Vickery. New York: Henry Holt, 1999.
- *Stretching,* by Bob Anderson. Bolinas, Calif.: Shelter Publications, 2000.

STRENGTH TRAINING

To read more about strength training, I recommend two excellent books.

- *Strength Training Past 50,* by Wayne Westcott. Champaign, Ill.: Human Kinetics Publications, 1997.

■ *Strong Women, Strong Bones,* by Miriam E. Nelson. New York: Putnam, 2000; www.strongwomen.com.

NUTRITION AND HEALTHFUL EATING

The following sites offer basic nutrition information, low-fat and vegetarian recipes, and, on the American Dietetic Association site, help in finding a registered dietitian in your area.

■ The American Dietetic Association: www.eatright.org
■ *Cooking Light* magazine: www.cookinglight.com
■ Low-Fat Vegetarian Recipe Archive: www.fatfree.com
■ Tufts University Nutrition Navigator: www.navigator.tufts.edu

If you select just one book on nutrition, I recommend this one.

■ *The Tufts University Guide to Total Nutrition,* by Stanley N. Gershoff et al. New York: HarperPerennial, 1996.

WEIGHT LOSS AND WEIGHT MANAGEMENT

These Web sites offer excellent nutrition guidance, helpful eating plans, and support for losing weight and maintaining a healthy weight.

■ The American Dietetic Association: www.eatright.org
■ The National Heart, Lung, and Blood Institute: www.nhlbi.nih.gov

In addition, the DASH (Dietary Approaches to Stop Hypertension) Diet, which in scientific tests proved very effective in helping to lower high blood pressure, can be used in a weight-loss program. The eating plan reduces intake of total and saturated fat and emphasizes fruits and vegetables. You can check out the diet at http://dash.bwh.harvard.edu. The National Heart, Lung, and Blood Institute also has information about the DASH Diet on its site (see above), or you can write to its information center at PO Box 30105, Bethesda, MD 20824-0105.

The Oldways Preservation and Exchange Trust, in cooperation with the Harvard School of Public Health, has developed pyramid guides that offer healthy eating plans for vegetarian cuisines and traditional ethnic cuisines such as Asian, Mediterranean, and Latin American. These work very well for planning a both reduced-calorie diet and a healthful diet in general. The Web address is www.oldwayspt.org.

The following books from the American Dietetic Association are also very helpful.

- *The American Dietetic Association's Complete Food and Nutrition Guide,* by Roberta Larson Duyff. New York: John Wiley, 1996.
- *Dieting for Dummies,* by Jane Kirby. Foster City, Calif.: IDG Books, 1998.

SUPPLEMENTS AND SUPPLEMENTATION

Almost every manufacturer or packager of supplements has a Web site to attract you to its products. How do you distinguish the potentially useful from the useless and even dangerous? In addition to the excellent book from the Arthritis Foundation listed below, you may want to check SupplementWatch at www.supplementwatch.com. This site provides independent, balanced reviews of most supplements by registered dietitians and other scientists.

ALTERNATIVE THERAPIES

The Arthritis Foundation has published a very good, balanced book that looks at all aspects of alternative and complementary approaches to arthritis. You can order it online at www.arthritis.org or by calling (800) 207-8633.

- *The Arthritis Foundation's Guide to Alternative Therapies,* by Judith Horstman. Atlanta, Ga.: Arthritis Foundation, 1999.

CLINICAL CLASSIFICATION CRITERIA FOR OSTEOARTHRITIS

Here are samples of the American College of Rheumatology (ACR) clinical classification criteria that physicians use when diagnosing osteoarthritis in three joints—the knee, hip, and hand. To see additional ACR classification criteria, visit the Johns Hopkins Arthritis Web site at www.hopkins-arthritis.com.jhmi.edu.

OSTEOARTHRITIS OF THE KNEE

Using patient history and physical examination:

Pain in the knee

and three of the following

Over 50 years of age
Less than 30 minutes of morning stiffness
Crepitus (crackling sound) on active motion
Bony tenderness
Bony enlargement
No palpable warmth of synovium

Using patient history, physical examination, and radiographic (x-ray) findings:

Pain in the knee

and one of the following

Over 50 years of age
Less than 30 minutes of morning stiffness
Crepitus (crackling sound) on active motion and
radiographic osteophytes (bony growths)

Using patient history, physical examination, and laboratory findings:

Pain in the knee

and five of the following

Over 50 years of age
Less than 30 minutes of morning stiffness
Crepitus (crackling sound) on active motion
Bony tenderness
Bony enlargement
No palpable warmth of synovium
ESR* less than 40mm/hr
Rheumatoid factor (RF) less than 1:40
Synovial fluid (SF) signs of osteoarthritis

OSTEOARTHRITIS OF THE HIP

Using patient history, physical examination, and laboratory findings:

Pain in the hip

and

Internal hip rotation less than 15°	**or**	Internal hip rotation more than 15°
and		**and**
ESR* less than 45mm/hr or hip flexion less than 115° if ESR is unavailable		Pain associated with internal hip
		and
		Less than 60 minutes of morning stiffness
		and
		Over 50 years of age

Using patient history, physical examination, laboratory, and radiographic (x-ray) findings:

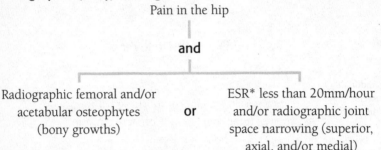

Pain in the hip

and

| Radiographic femoral and/or acetabular osteophytes (bony growths) | **or** | ESR* less than 20mm/hour and/or radiographic joint space narrowing (superior, axial, and/or medial) |

OSTEOARTHRITIS OF THE HAND

Pain, aching, or stiffness in the hand

and three of the following

Hard-tissue enlargement of two or more of the following joints: 2nd and 3rd distal interphalangeal; 2nd and 3rd proximal interphalangeal; 1st carpometacarpal joints of both hands

Hard-tissue enlargement of two or more distal interphalangeal joints

Less than three swollen metacarpal joints

Deformity of at least one of the following joints: 2nd and 3rd distal interphalangeal; 2nd and 3rd proximal interphalangeal; 1st carpometacarpal joints of both hands

---

*ESR stands for erythrocyte sedimentation rate; elevated sedimentation rates indicate the presence of inflammation.

INDEX

Level 3 upper-body exercises in, 106–7, 108
maintenance after, 108
8-Week Stretching Program. *See also* Stretching
equipment for, 86
general guidelines for, 86–87
Level 1 stretches in, 87, 88–89, 92–94
Level 2 stretches in, 90–91, 94–95
Level 3 stretches in, 92–93, 95–96
maintenance after, 96
8-Week Walking Program. *See also* Walking
components of, 64
equipment for, 60–61
levels of
green, 67
red, 65–66
yellow, 66–67
overview of, 64–65
principles of effective exercise in, 62–64
Elimination diets, 127–28
Equipment
sports, choosing, 174
for strength training, 99
for stretching, 86
for walking, 60–61
Examination, joint, by physician, 145–46
Exercise. *See also specific exercises*
aerobic (*see* Aerobic exercise)
effective, principles of, 62–64
for ending and preventing joint pain, 15–16
injuries from, preventing, 60, 173–74
resources for, 180–81
weight loss and 115, 116, 117

F

Fasting, avoiding, 126–27
Fat, dietary
limiting, for joint health, 120
unhealthful vs. healthful, 122–23, 141
50-foot walk test, 41, 42

Fingers
dexterity program for, 108–10
pain in, evaluating, 36–37
Finger stretch, 109
Finger-to-thumb touch, 109
advanced, 110
Fish oil, as supplement, 134–35
Flaxseed, as supplement, 135
Flexibility
benefits of, 84
from stretching program (*see* 8-Week Stretching Program)
Fractures, 172
Front arm circles, 94
Front arm raises, 87

G

Gardening
health benefits of, 71, 73–75
locations for, 77
safety guidelines for, 77–78
seasonal activities in, 75–77
Gelatin-based supplements
findings on, 23
in joint health study, 18, 19–20
overview of, 131–32
recommendations for, 137, 141, 167
General health
activity for benefiting, 72–73
effect of aging on, 163
resources for, 180
Glucosamine, as supplement, 132–33, 137, 141
Gout
foods, as triggers for, 121
low-purine diet for, 124

H

Hands
dexterity program for, 108–10
osteoarthritis of, classification criteria for, 186

W

X

ABOUT THE AUTHOR

Dr. James Rippe is founder and director of the Rippe Lifestyle Institute in Shrewsbury, Massachusetts; founder and director of Rippe Health Assessment at Celebration Health in Celebration, Florida; and associate professor of medicine (cardiology) at Tufts University School of Medicine in Boston.

Dr. Rippe is regarded as one of the leading authorities in the United States on preventive cardiology, health and fitness, and healthy weight loss. Under his leadership, the Rippe Lifestyle Institute has conducted many research projects on the impact of positive lifestyle choices on good health and quality of life.

Dr. Rippe has written 25 books, including 15 medical texts and 10 books on health and fitness for the general public, including *Fitness Walking*, *The Sports Performance Factors*, *Fitness Walking for Women*, *Fit for Success*, *The Rockport Walking Program*, *The Complete Book of Fitness Walking*, *The Exercise Exchange Program*, *Fit over Forty*, *The Healthy Heart for Dummies*, and *The Healthy Heart Cookbook for Dummies*. His most recent medical textbook, *Lifestyle Medicine*, is a comprehensive guide for physicians on the impact of lifestyle choices on health.

A lifelong athlete, Dr. Rippe maintains his personal fitness with a regular walking, jogging, and weight-training program. He holds a black belt in karate and is an avid wind surfer, skier, and tennis player. He lives near Boston with his wife, television news anchor Stephanie Hart, and their four children, Hart, Jaelin, Devon, and Jamie.